Handbook of
Eczema
for Practitioners

Kabir Sardana MD DNB MNAMS
Professor
Department of Dermatology
Maulana Azad Medical College
and Lok Nayak Hospital
New Delhi

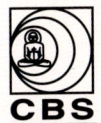

CBS Publishers & Distributors Pvt Ltd

New Delhi • Bengaluru • Chennai • Kochi • Kolkata • Mumbai
Hyderabad • Nagpur • Patna • Pune • Vijayawada

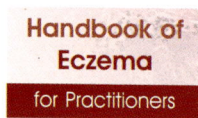

Handbook of Eczema
for Practitioners

ISBN: 978-93-85915-05-5 (Soft Cover)

ISBN: 978-93-85915-06-2 (Hard Cover)

Copyright © Author and Publisher

First Edition: 2016

Published by Satish Kumar Jain and produced by Varun Jain for

CBS Publishers & Distributors Pvt Ltd

4819/XI Prahlad Street, 24 Ansari Road, Daryaganj, New Delhi 110 002, India.

Ph: 23289259, 23266861, 23266867 Website: www.cbspd.com

Fax: 011-23243014   e-mail: delhi@cbspd.com; cbspubs@airtelmail.in.

Corporate Office: 204 FIE, Industrial Area, Patparganj, Delhi 110 092

Ph: 4934 4934   Fax: 4934 4935   e-mail: publishing@cbspd.com; publicity@cbspd.com

Branches

- **Bengaluru:** Seema House 2975, 17th Cross, K.R. Road, Banasankari 2nd Stage, Bengaluru 560 070, Karnataka
  Ph: +91-80-26771678/79   Fax: +91-80-26771680   e-mail: bangalore@cbspd.com
- **Chennai:** 7, Subbaraya Street, Shenoy Nagar, Chennai 600 030, Tamil Nadu
  Ph: +91-44-26680620, 26681266   Fax: +91-44-42032115   e-mail: chennai@cbspd.com
- **Kochi:** Ashana House, No. 39/1904, AM Thomas Road, Valanjambalam, Ernakulam 682 018, Kochi, Kerala
  Ph: +91-484-4059061-65   Fax: +91-484-4059065   e-mail: kochi@cbspd.com
- **Kolkata:** 6/B, Ground Floor, Rameswar Shaw Road, Kolkata-700 014, West Bengal
  Ph: +91-33-22891126, 22891127, 22891128   e-mail: kolkata@cbspd.com
- **Mumbai:** 83-C, Dr E Moses Road, Worli, Mumbai-400018, Maharashtra
  Ph: +91-22-24902340/41   Fax: +91-22-24902342   e-mail: mumbai@cbspd.com

Representatives

- **Hyderabad** 0-9885175004
- **Nagpur** 0-9021734563
- **Patna** 0-9334159340
- **Pune** 0-9623451994
- **Vijayawada** 0-9000660880

Printed at Magic International, Greater Noida

to

---

my wife Dr Supriya Mahajan, the philosopher-guide and the veritable "Rock of Gibraltor", who has stood by me through thick and thin

my daughter Zoya, the epitome of godliness

my parents Amba Sardana and Maj Gen KN Sardana, Dehradun, who are luckily far away from the rat race

my teachers and students

I also dedicate this book to some unique people who have been a source of inspiration, encouragement and support in recent times; people who defy the commonly held belief that good people are a rarity

Shri Rajiv Aggarwal, who is like a father figure to me

Dr RP Gupta, a man of few words but with a heart of Gold

Dr Arun Gupta, for whom it can be said "God helps those who help others"

and

Shri Anil Kumar Sharma, former RTI Commissioner, Uttaranchal

Don't wait for great things to happen. Great things do happen, but don't wait for something great to happen. It happens only when you start living small, ordinary, day-to-day things, with a new mind, vitality, freshness and enthusiasm. Then, by and by you accumulate and one day that explodes into sheer joy.

Most of us miss this because we are waiting for something great to happen. It can't happen, it only happens through small things: eating your breakfast, walking, lying on the grass, talking to a friend, just sitting alone, meditating, looking at the sky or just lying on the bed doing nothing.

These are the small things that life is made of, they are the very stuff of life.

and

The day you decide not to ask for things that you like, but rather to like things that happen, that day you become mature.

—**OSHO**

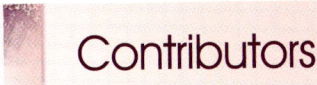

Contributors

Aniket Bhole
Secondary DNB, Hindu Rao Hospital, Delhi, *Chapter 8*

Chia-Chun Ang MBBS (Singapore), MRCP (UK), MMed (Int Med), FAMS (Dermatology)
Consultant Dermatologist, Changi General Hospital, Singapore, *Chapter 9*

Deepshikha Khanna MD (Dermatology)
Consultant (Specialist), Dermatology
Lal Bahadur Shastri Hospital
Mayur Vihar, Khichripur
Delhi 110091, *Chapter 7*

Khushbu Mahajan MD
Assistant Professor, North Delhi Municipal Corporation Medical College and Hindu
Rao Hospital, Delhi, *Chapter 8*

Sanjay Ghosh
Professor, Department of Dermatology
MGM Medical College and LSK Hospital
Kishanganj, India, *Chapter 6*

Saurav Kundu
Assistant Professor, Department of Dermatology
MGM Medical College and LSK Hospital
Kishanganj, India, *Chapter 6*

Shivani Bansal MD, DNB
Max Panchsheel, Delhi, *Chapters 5, 11, 12, 17, 20*

Soumya Agarwal
Senior Resident, Department of Dermatology, Lady Hardinge Medical College and
SSKH, Delhi, *Chapter 3*

Taru Garg
Professor, Department of Dermatology, Lady Hardinge Medical College and
SSKH, Delhi, *Chapter 3*

Wai-Kwong Cheong MBBS (Singapore), MRCP (UK), FRCP (Edinburgh), FAMS (Dermatology)
Consultant Dermatologist, Specialist Skin Clinic and Associates, Singapore,
Chapter 9

Foreword

It gives me immense pleasure to write the Foreword to this book, *Handbook of Eczema for Practitioners*, which is written by an academic champion as well as a clinician extraordinaire. Prof Kabir Sardana holds an excellent academic record, has numerous research publications of prime quality in journals of international repute and is a splendid teacher of dermatology.

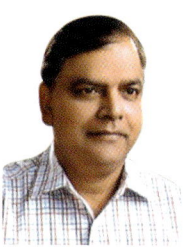

The term 'Eczema' encompasses a gamut of unrelated dermatological conditions causing inflammation of the skin. Eczemas form a significant bulk of dermatology practice. Often, we see inappropriately managed patients of eczema due to unavailability of dermatologists at medical facilities of first contact. Unfortunately, not much dermatology is taught in MBBS curriculum. I daresay, there is scarcity in understanding of dermatologic disease patterns among general and family physicians. There are very few books specifically dealing with eczemas across the world and even fewer in India.

This treatise should go a long way in fulfilling this unmet need. The USP of this book is its simplicity and stress on clinical recognition of different conditions. This handbook is of great value to practicing dermatologists, general and family physicians, dermatologic nurses as well as PG students. In addition to providing detailed knowledge of different conditions, this book is also an effective ready-reckoner for eczemas in any clinical setting. I congratulate Prof Sardana and all the authors for this valuable contribution to our field and I hope this book finds all the popularity that it so truly deserves.

RP Gupta
Consultant Dermatologist
Delhi

Preface

Eczema is probably one of the most commonly seen skin disorders but there is probably just one book dedicated to it on the Fast Fact Series. In Asian skin the manifestations and causes are different than in the West. The aim of this book was to succinctly cover the major types of eczema focusing on Indian and Asian skin.

A book is worth its contributors and I am fortunate to have contributors who have special interest in their respective topics. **Dr Sanjay Ghosh** has extensive experience in airborne contact dermatitis, a major problem in India. **Dr Taru Garg** has done work on allergic contact dermatitis which in India is massive problem as the number of allergens outmaneuver the tools and I daresay the clinicians to identify them. **Dr Deepshikha Khanna** had worked for many years in an exclusive pediatric dermatology set up and contributes on diaper dermatitis. **Dr Pooja Arora Mrig** has interest in a difficult and recurring problem of hand eczema, a issue in India, where the majority of housewives who are exposed to ever strong detergents promoted by the media and are consequentially plagued by this problem. **Dr Khushbu Mahajan** has an interest in atopic dermatitis, a condition that in the humid weather of the country is still largely a manageable disorder. **Dr Wai-Kwong Cheong** has done extensive work on seborrheic eczema, a condition that is common in the humid environment that is seen both In India and Singapore. Lastly **Dr Shivani Bansal** has done justice to the other topics that encompass the commonly see eczematous disorders.

The book is not aimed to be a treatise and thus we have purposely left out the verbose pathogenesis and focused on the clinical approach and management concept of this dermatological series that had been supported by CBS Publishers.

Lastly a big thanks to the team at CBS, Mr SK Jain (Matta), CMD, Mr YN Arjuna, Sr Vice President, Mrs Ritu Chawla, Mr SK Verma and Mr Sunil Dutt and the great support staff of artists and proofreaders at their office.

Happy reading!

Kabir Sardana

Contents

Contributors	*vii*
Foreword by RP Gupta	*ix*
Preface	*xi*

1. Introduction — 1
2. Irritant Eczema — 8
3. Allergic Contact Eczema — 17
4. Non-Eczematous Contact Dermatitis — 39
5. Photoallergic Eczema — 47
6. Airborne Contact Dermatitis — 56
7. Diaper Dermatitis — 66
8. Atopic Dermatitis — 77
9. Seborrheic Eczema — 98
10. Asteatotic Eczema — 107
11. Discoid Eczema — 109
12. Pityriasis Alba — 114
13. Hand Eczema — 119
14. Hyperkeratotic Eczema of the Palms — 134
15. Acute and Recurrent Vesicular Hand Eczema (Syn Pompholyx) — 138
16. Juvenile Plantar Dermatosis — 143
17. Venous Eczema — 145
18. Lichen Simplex Chronicus — 149
19. Exfoliative Erythroderma — 154
20. Prurigo Nodularis — 158

Index — *165*

Introduction

INTRODUCTION

Eczemas are probably the most common skin condition seen by family physicians. While being a disparate group of diseases, they have some common features including the presence of itch and in the acute stages, edema (spongiosis) in the epidermis. In early disease the stratum corneum remains intact, so the eczema appears as a red smooth edematous plaque. With worsening disease the edema becomes more severe, tense blisters appear. If less severe or if the eczema becomes chronic, scaling and epithelial disruption occurs, giving chronic eczema the characteristic appearance. All these are phases of the reaction pattern and are known as eczema. The word eczema comes from the Greek for 'boiling'—a reference to the tiny vesicles (bubbles) that are often seen in the early acute stages of the disorder, but less often in its later chronic stages. Dermatitis means inflammation of the skin and is therefore, strictly speaking, a broader term than eczema—which is just one of several possible types of skin inflammation.

Though various classification exist we will stick to the the time-honoured, division into exogenous and endogenous types (Table 1.1).

In this book we will discuss the common types of eczema and the rare variants will be left to specialized dermatology textbooks.

Stages of Eczema

There are three stages of eczema: Acute, subacute, and chronic (Fig. 1.1). Clinically, an eczematous disease may start at any stage and evolve into another. We will give detail of the various types and their treatment.

Table 1.1: Classification of eczema

Exogenous eczemas

- Irritant eczema
- Allergic contact eczema
- Photoallergic eczema
- ABCD
- Eczematous polymorphic light eruption
- Infective eczema
- Dermatophytide
- Post-traumatic eczema

Endogenous eczema

- Atopic eczema
- Seborrheic eczema
- Asteatotic eczema
- Discoid eczema
- Eyelid eczema
- Exudative discoid and lichenoid chronic dermatosis
- Chronic superficial scaly dermatitis
- Pityriasis alba
- Hand eczema
- Venous eczema
- Juvenile plantar dermatosis
- Eczematous drug eruptions
- Lichen simplex chronicus
- Prurigo nodularis

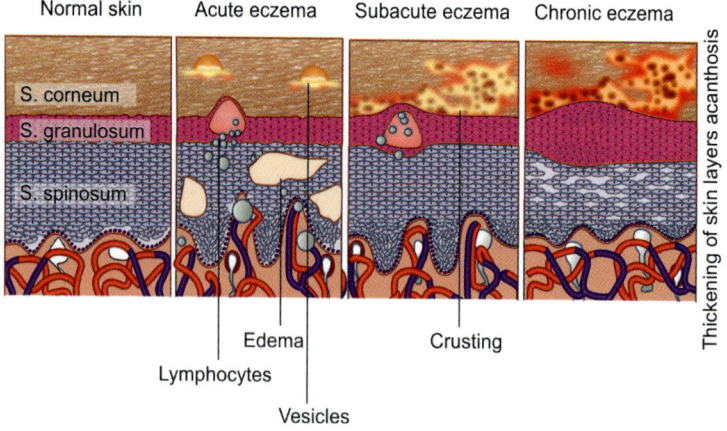

Fig. 1.1: A depiction of the phases of eczema

1. Acute Eczema

Etiology. Inflammation is caused by contact with specific allergens such as Rhus (poison ivy, oak, or sumac) and chemicals. In the id reaction, vesicular reactions occur at a distant site during or after a fungal infection, stasis dermatitis, or other acute inflammatory processes (Fig. 1.2).

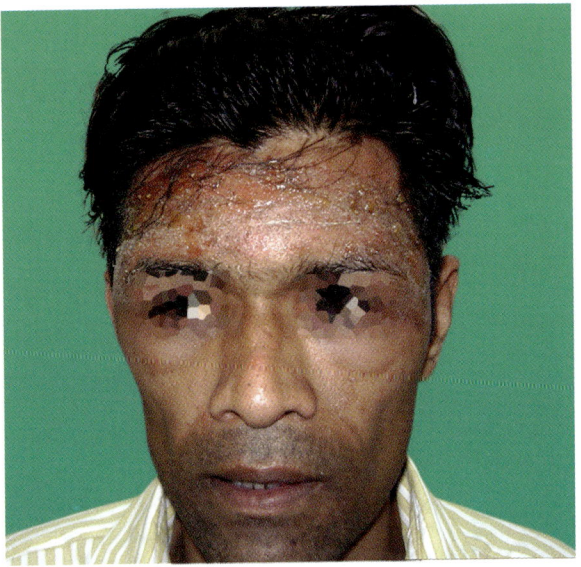

Fig. 1.2: A case of acute eczema in a patient consequent to allergic contact dermatitis to hair dye

Clinical Findings

The classic features are:
1. Weeping and crusting
2. Blistering—usually with vesicles
3. Redness, papules and swelling—usually with an ill-defined border; and
4. Scaling.

There is frequently intense itching and heat and hot water can accentuate the symptoms. The condition can persist for a week or more and can evolve into a subacute stage before resolving.

Treatment

1. *Cool, wet dressings.* The evaporative cooling produced by wet compresses causes vasoconstriction and rapidly suppresses inflammation and itching. Either Burow's solution or normal saline can be used. A clean cotton cloth is soaked in cool water, folded several times, and placed directly over the affected areas. Evaporative cooling produces vasoconstriction and decreases serum production. Wet compresses should **not** be held in place and covered with towels or plastic wrap because this prevents evaporation. The wet cloth macerates vesicles and, when removed, mechanically debrides the area and prevents serum and crust from accumulating. Wet compresses should be removed after 30 minutes and replaced with a freshly soaked cloth.

2. *Oral corticosteroids.* Oral corticosteroids such as prednisone are useful for controlling intense or widespread inflammation and may be used in addition to wet dressings. A course of 20 mg dose twice or once a day for 7 to 14 days is enough in most cases though is some cases up to 21 days of therapy may be needed. Topical corticosteroids are of a little use in the acute stage because the cream does not penetrate through the vesicles.

3. *Antihistamines.* Antihistamines, relieve itching and provide enough sedation so patients can sleep.

4. *Antibiotics.* The use of oral antibiotics may greatly hasten resolution of the disease if signs of superficial secondary infection, are present. Cephalexin and dicloxacillin are effective.

2. Subacute Eczema

There is erythema and scaling with an indistinct border (Fig. 1.3). The symptoms vary from no itching to intense itching. Subacute eczematous inflammation may be the initial stage or it may follow acute inflammation. If the inciting agent is withdrawn, the condition often resolves but excessive drying created from washing or continued use of wet dressings causes cracking and fissures (Fig. 1.3).

Treatment

It is important to discontinue wet dressings when acute inflammation evolves into subacute inflammation. Excess drying creates cracking and fissures, which predispose to infection.

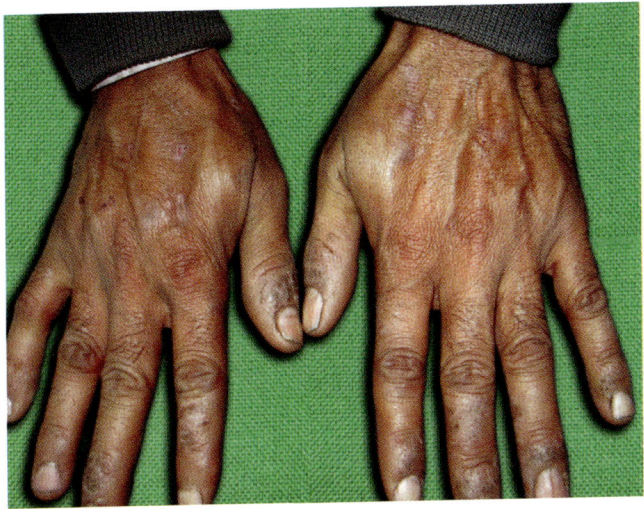

Fig. 1.3: A case of contact dermatitis to cement a prototype of subacute eczema

1. Topical Corticosteroids. These agents are the treatment of choice.
2. Topical Macrolide Immune Suppressants. Tacrolimus ointment and pimecrolimus cream have been used for atopic dermatitis, allergic contact dermatitis, and irritant contact dermatitis and are approved for use in children 2 years or older. Response to these agents is slower than the response to topical steroids.
3. Lubrication. This is a simple but essential part of therapy. Inflamed skin becomes dry and is more susceptible to further irritation and inflammation. Resolved dry areas may easily relapse into subacute eczema if proper lubrication is neglected. They can be applied a few hours *after* topical steroids and should be continued for days or weeks after the inflammation has cleared. Frequent application (one to four times a day) should be encouraged and using them after the skin has been patted dry following a shower seals in moisture.
4. Mild Soaps. Frequent washing with a drying soap, can be avoided by using superfatted soaps.
5. Antibiotics. Eczematous plaques that remain bright red during treatment with topical steroids may be infected. Infected subacute eczema should be treated with appropriate systemic

antibiotics, which are usually those active against Staphylococci. Systemic antibiotics are more effective than topical antibiotics or antibiotic-steroid combination creams.

3. Chronic Eczema

Chronic eczematous inflammation may be caused by irritation of subacute inflammation, or it may appear as lichen simplex chronicus (Fig. 1.4). Chronic eczematous inflammation is a clinical-pathologic entity and does not indicate simply any long-lasting stage of eczema. If scratching is not controlled, subacute eczematous inflammation can be modified and converted to chronic eczematous inflammation.

There is moderate to intense itching. Scratching sometimes becomes violent, leading to excoriation and digging, and ceases only when pain has replaced the itch. Patients with chronic inflammation scratch while asleep. They are:

1. Less vesicular and exudative.
2. More scaly, pigmented and thickened.
3. More likely to show lichenification—a dry leathery thickened state, with increased skin markings, secondary to repeated scratching or rubbing.
4. More likely to fissure.

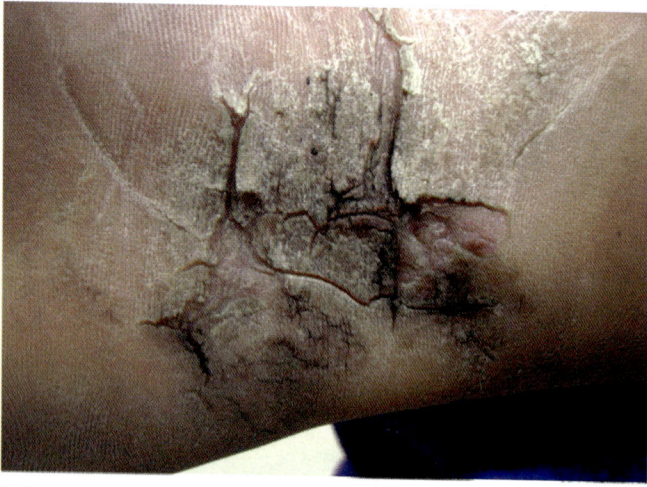

Fig. 1.4: A case of hyperkeratotic eczema, a prototype of chronic eczema

Treatment

Chronic eczematous inflammation is resistant to treatment and requires potent steroid therapy.

Intralesional Injection. Intralesional injection is a very effective mode of therapy. Lesions that have been present for years may completely resolve after one injection or a short series of injections. The medicine is delivered with a 27- or 30-gauge needle, and the entire plaque is infiltrated until it blanches white. Resistant plaques require additional injections given at 3- to 4-week intervals.

Bibliography

1. Eczema, in. Sardana k, Mahajan S, Garg VK. Diagnosis and Management of Skin Disorders: An Evidence-Based Approach, 1/e.: Lippincott Williams and Wilkins, 2012 (reprint 2015).
2. Fast Facts: Eczema and Contact Dermatitis By John Berth-Jones, Eunice Tan and Howard I Malbach Published 2004.
3. Thieme Clinical Companions Dermatology. Sterry, Dermatology© 2006 Thieme.

2

Irritant Eczema

IRRITANT CONTACT DERMATITIS (ICD)

Exogenous eczemas can be irritant or allergic. They are diagnosed predominantly on the distribution, which suggests contact with a precipitating factor. Irritant eczemas are a result of agents that produce keratinocyte damage without immunological memory.

Irritant Contact Dermatitis ICD: This accounts for more than 80% of all cases of contact dermatitis, and most of the cases are from factories. Though most commonly they involve the hand, they can also be seen in children (e.g. as a reaction to a bubble bath, play dough or lip-licking).

A working classification of ICD is given in Box 2.1.

Box 2.1: Classification of irritant contact dermatitis	
Phases	Acute irritant contact dermatitis Cumulative irritant contact dermatitis
Variants	Lip lick dermatitis Ring dermatitis Wear and tear dermatitis Finger tip dermatitis Diaper dermatitis

Cause

Strong irritants elicit an acute reaction after brief contact and the diagnosis is then usually obvious. Prolonged exposure, sometimes over years, is needed for weak irritants to cause dermatitis, usually of the hands and forearms. Water, detergents, chemicals, solvents, cutting oils and abrasive dusts are common culprits. Other causes include frequent use of soaps and detergents, exposure to organic or alkaline solvents, exposure to an environment with low humidity, or chronic exposure to saliva (lip lick dermatitis), urine, or feces. There is a wide range of susceptibility with those with very dry skin being especially vulnerable. Past or present atopic dermatitis doubles the risk of irritant hand eczema. Areas where the water is "hard" tend to have a higher prevalence of ICD due to the potential "drying " effect of hard water. The irritant effect of water is an intriguing phenomenon. The overhydration of the skin in wet-work occupations not only enhances the penetration of many irritants but may also release inflammatory mediators *and their inhibitors* from the stratum corneum, the mechanism of which may lead to a gradual damage of the skin.

Recently, the SLS test has been used in patch testing as a way of differentiating between allergic and irritant reactions. If SLS reacts during patch testing, it is likely that macular, erythematous reactions to patch test samples have an irritant etiology. On the other hand, if the skin does not react to SLS, it is likely that these reactions to allergens during patch testing are allergic in etiology. Although the SLS can be helpful, it is very important to keep in mind that it is impossible to correlate results with every possible irritant agent.

Clinical Features

1. Acute Irritant CD

This is caused by a single sudden exposure to a irritant and caustic chemical and is characterized by burning, pain, edema, intense vesiculation with frequent sloughing of the exposed part (Fig. 2.1). In case of exposure to a liquid agent, a dripping of the liquid is evident as a skin reaction.

2.Cumulative ICD

This is caused by repeated exposure to an allergen and most frequently affects the dorsal aspect of the hand, finger webs, face and eyelids. Most cases are seen in housewives where it is called "**housewives dermatitis or dish pan hands or detergent hands**. Other occupations affected include mothers with young children (e.g. from changing diapers), individuals whose jobs require repeated wetting and drying (e.g. surgeons, dentists, dishwashers, bartenders, fishermen), industrial workers whose jobs require

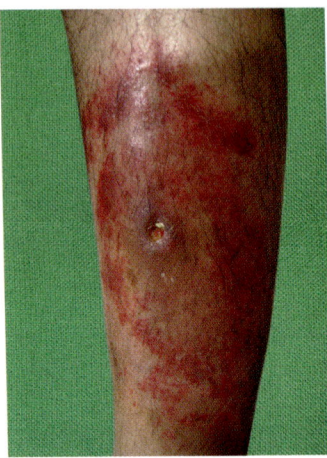

Fig. 2.1: A intense ICD (irritant contact dermatitis) due to the use of betadine (povidone iodine) around a leg ulcer

contact with chemicals (e.g. cutting oils), and patients with the atopic diathesis.

Pathogenesis: The stratum corneum is the protective envelope that prevents exogenous material from entering the skin and prevents body water from escaping. The stratum corneum of the palms is thicker than that of the backs of the hands and is more resistant to irritation. The pH of this surface layer is slightly acidic. Environmental factors or elements that change any component of the stratum corneum interfere with its protective function and expose the skin to irritants. These include hard water, cold winter air, hot water, harsh soaps and low humidity. This repeated insult leads to a higher predisposition to developing eczema.

Clinical findings

Dryness and chapping is the initial changes, this is followed by painful cracks and fissures. The backs of the hands become red, swollen, and tender. The palmar surface, especially that of the fingers, becomes red and continues to be dry and cracked (Fig. 2.2).

Differential diagnosis

The differentiation of cumulative irritant contact dermatitis from another dermatitic process or an eczematous lesion of the skin is a challenge.

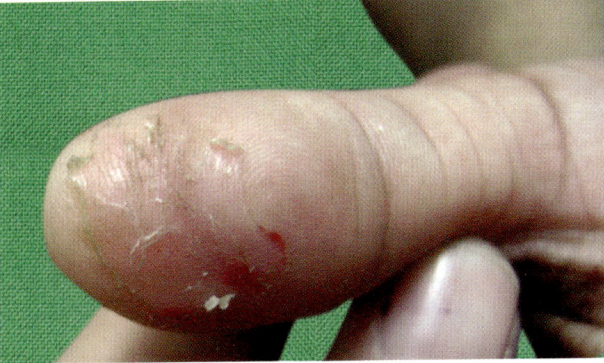

Fig. 2.2: A case of cumulative ICD in a housewife localized on the fingertips, primarily due to a combination of detergent use and cutting vegetables

a. *Atopic dermatitis* often occurs on the hands in young adults and is provoked and aggravated in occupations with a high exposure to water and irritants, such as hairdressing, cleaning, and housekeeping. It is often difficult to weigh the individual role of irritants and atopic constitution. In many cases, it is the atopic disorder of the skin that is primarily responsible for the development of a cumulative irritant contact dermatitis.

b. *Psoriasis* of the hands can imitate eczema or an irritant contact dermatitis. Careful examination of the whole skin to look for minor signs of psoriasis is important. In the follow-up of these patients, psoriasis may develop in other areas. Sometimes a combination of atopy and psoriasis occurs on the hands with itchy vesicles. Some of these patients experience a sudden aggravation of the dermatitis after exposure to water.

c. *Tinea of the hands* may simulate a dry palmar dermatitis. Unilateral localization and involvement of the nails are important clues to diagnose tinea.

d. Prolonged exposure to organic solvents may cause scaly, hyperkeratotic skin on the palmar side of the hands, which has to be differentiated from the *hyperkeratotic palmar eczema* (tylotic eczema). Irritants and allergens may complicate hyperkeratotic eczema, another endogenous dermatosis with features of psoriasis and eczema.

e. The differentiation between a cumulative irritant and an allergic contact dermatitis is a great challenge but not often possible

(Fig. 2.3). In general, an allergic contact dermatitis is more *polymorphic*, with an *unsharp* demarcation, with a tendency for *spreading*, and with occasional localizations at the wrist, the forearm, and the face, especially on the eyelids. The course is often relapsing, with improvement during weekends and holidays. In the work environment, only one or a few persons are affected, and a relevant positive patch test makes the diagnosis definitive.

Especially in the case of fingertip dermatitis and eczema, it is impossible to differentiate an allergic contact dermatitis from a cumulative irritant contact dermatitis or psoriasis. Long-standing cases of allergic contact dermatitis with a lichenoid character (nickel and chromate allergies) may change in character from eczematous to more psoriasis-like.

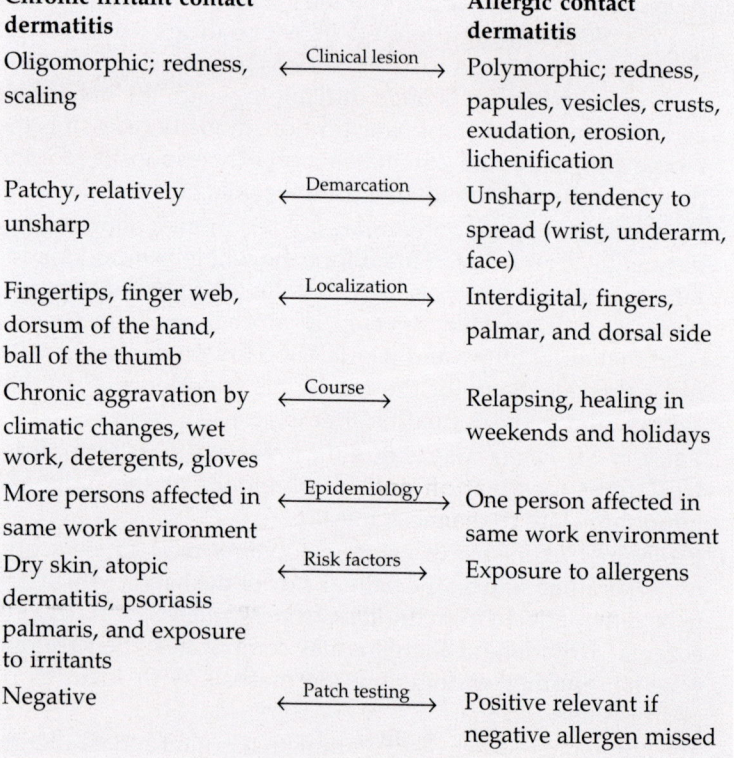

Chronic irritant contact dermatitis		Allergic contact dermatitis
Oligomorphic; redness, scaling	← Clinical lesion →	Polymorphic; redness, papules, vesicles, crusts, exudation, erosion, lichenification
Patchy, relatively unsharp	← Demarcation →	Unsharp, tendency to spread (wrist, underarm, face)
Fingertips, finger web, dorsum of the hand, ball of the thumb	← Localization →	Interdigital, fingers, palmar, and dorsal side
Chronic aggravation by climatic changes, wet work, detergents, gloves	← Course →	Relapsing, healing in weekends and holidays
More persons affected in same work environment	← Epidemiology →	One person affected in same work environment
Dry skin, atopic dermatitis, psoriasis palmaris, and exposure to irritants	← Risk factors →	Exposure to allergens
Negative	← Patch testing →	Positive relevant if negative allergen missed

Fig. 2.3: A depiction of the differences between chronic ICD and ACD

Treatment

The simplest method is by prevention of allergen and the use of an emulsion cleanser (e.g. Cetaphil lotion) can lead to a marked decrease in dryness and eczema.

Barrier-Protectant Creams. Loss of skin barrier function by mechanical or chemical insults may result in water loss and hand eczema. Barrier creams applied at least twice a day on all exposed areas protect the skin and are formulated to be either water-repellent or oil-repellent. The water-repellent types offer a little protection against oils or solvents.

The inflammation is similar to principles of treating subacute eczema. Lubrication and avoidance of further irritation help to prevent recurrence (Table 2.1).

3. Lip Lick Dermatitis

This is a common variant seen in children and is consequent to licking of the lips and is usually periorificial in distribution (Fig. 2.4) and is usually complicated by secondary infection and contact allergy due to the use of topical medicaments.

Table 2.1: A list of common methods to avoid recurrence

a. Wash hands as infrequently as possible. Ideally, soap should be avoided and hands simply washed in lukewarm water.

b. Shampooing must be done with rubber gloves or by someone else.

c. Avoid direct contact with household cleaners and detergents. Wear cotton, plastic, or rubber gloves when doing housework. A sensible option is to use cotton gloves under rubber gloves.

d. Do not touch or do not do anything that causes burning or itching (e.g. wool; wet diapers; peeling potatoes or handling fresh fruits, vegetables, and raw meat).

e. Wear rubber gloves when irritants are encountered. Rubber gloves alone are not sufficient because the lining collects sweat, scales, and debris and can become more irritating than those objects to be avoided. Dermal white cotton gloves should be worn next to the skin under unlined rubber gloves. Several pairs of cotton gloves should be purchased so they can be changed frequently. Ensure the rubber gloves fit comfortably over the white cotton gloves.

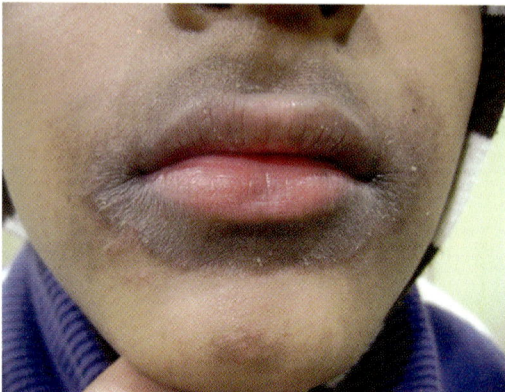

Fig. 2.4: A case of lip lick dermatitis in a school going child aggravated due to exam stress

4. Ring Dermatitis

This is seen in females after marriage and in this there is a patch of eczema that begins around the wedding ring (Fig. 2.5). This is due to three factors, trapping of detergent under the ring, friction and trauma. The eczema patch frequently extends beyond the involved finger to involve the middle finger and adjacent palm.

Removing the ring while working is one of the simplest ways to avoid this type of eczema.

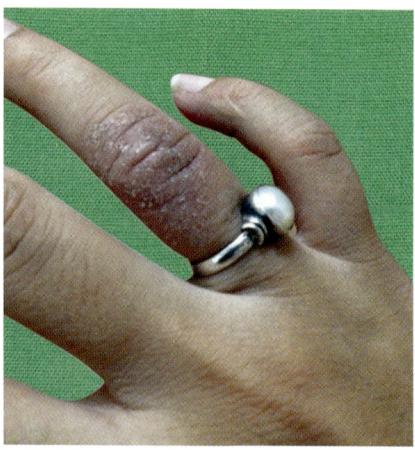

Fig. 2.5: A case of ring eczema in a newly married patient due to the use of detergents

5. Wear and Tear Dermatitis

Again this is seen in housewives and cleaners and is characterized by sharply demarcated areas of thick scaling or hyperkeratosis on the palms (and frequently on the soles) (Fig. 2.6). The condition may be confused with psoriasis, but there is a little or none of the redness and none of the scaling or nail changes typical of psoriasis. The condition is more common in middle-aged and elderly persons and in men.

6. Fingertip Eczema

This may be due to both allergic contact dermatitis and irritant contact dermatitis. One finger or several fingers may be involved. Initially the skin may be moist and then may become dry, cracked, and scaly and when the skin peels from the fingertips distally, a dry, red, cracked, fissured, tender or painful surface without skin lines is revealed (Fig. 2.2). Once allergy and psoriasis have been ruled out, fingertip eczema should be managed the same way as subacute and chronic eczema—by avoiding irritants and lubricating frequently.

7. Diaper Dermatitis*

Though various causes can lead to diaper dermatitis, the most common is the irritant diaper dermatitis which is rare in the neonatal period but is common in the first 18 months of life.

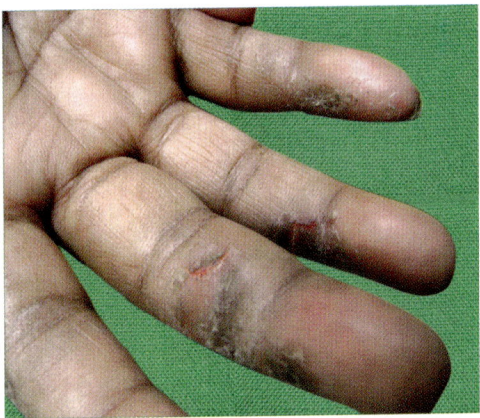

Fig. 2.6: Chronic eczema in a housewife, note the hyperkeratosis and fissuring in the involved areas

*Also see Chapter 7.

Irritant dermatitis is caused by exposure of the skin to feces and/or urine trapped in the diaper as infants are physiologically incontinent. Using absorbent diapers and changing the diaper frequently can limit the occurrence of irritant dermatitis.

The most commonly encountered clinical presentation is *erythema of the convex zones*. The bright red erythema covers the convex areas of the buttocks (in a W shape) and may spread to the pubis and upper thighs. It can become shiny and erosive with a corroded appearance.

Other, rarer forms of irritant dermatitis include:

The *pseudoverrucous papules* form, the *papulo-erosive* form (known as Sevestre and Jacquet erosive dermatitis), the *vesicular form (known as Parrot dermatitis)*, and the nodular form or *infantile gluteal granuloma*.

Treatment

The first-line treatment, where possible, is to eliminate the cause (cloth diapers, for example). Parents often feel guilty about diaper dermatitis which leads them to employ over-zealous hygiene measures and multiple topical treatments which ultimately aggravate the irritation. They must be reassured, told to be patient and given clear advice about how to care for the diaper area. The diaper should be changed frequently (>6/day), the area washed with a gentle detergent (soap-free detergent or a cleansing oil) and a barrier cream applied at least twice a day (especially those containing zinc and copper). A short course of topical corticosteroids can be prescribed to treat forms with papular lesions.

If the presence of *C. albicans* is suspected, particularly if there is no improvement after several days, a topical antifungal preparation may be used.

Bibliography

1. Eczema, in. Sardana k, Mahajan S, Garg VK. Diagnosis and Management of Skin Disorders: An Evidence-Based Approach, 1/ e.: Lippincott Williams and Wilkins, 2012 (reprint 2015).
2. Fast Facts: Eczema and Contact Dermatitis By John Berth-Jones, Eunice Tan and Howard I Malbach Published 2004.
3. Thieme Clinical Companions Dermatology. Sterry, Dermatology© 2006 Thieme.

Allergic Contact Eczema

ALLERGIC CONTACT DERMATITIS

The term 'allergie' was first coined by the scientist von Pirquet in 1906 (Adams RM, 1983). The word was derived from the Greek *allos* and *ergon*, meaning other or different work (Ayto J, 1990). Contact dermatitis accounts for 4–7% of all dermatological consultations. Of all contact dermatitis cases, around 20 percent are caused by allergic contact dermatitis (ACD). It represents the classic cutaneous presentation of delayed type hypersensitivity response to exogenous antigens.

Definition

ACD can be defined as a delayed type IV allergic reaction of the skin presenting with varying degrees of erythema, edema, and vesiculation resulting from cutaneous contact with a specific allergen.

Epidemiology

ACD affects approximately 7% of the general population (Heine G et al, 2004). An Indian study reported positive patch test reactions in 50% of the patients (Sharma VK et al, 2010). **Nickel sulphate** was the most common sensitizer (43.7%), followed by fragrance mix (18.6%), paraben mix, potassium dichromate, cobalt, and formaldehyde. Westernization of lifestyle in India has resulted in an increased exposure to cosmetics, hair and other dyes, and packaged food.

Pathogenesis

Allergic contact dermatitis involves two main processes of sensitization (afferent or induction phase), and elicitation (efferent or challenge phase) (Flow chart 3.1). The induction of sensitivity is the primary event which is initiated by binding of allergens to skin components, and association of these products with major histocompatibility complex (MHC) class II molecules (Lepoittevin J-P, 2006). These complete or conjugated antigens are recognised by T lymphocytes in the presence of other co-stimulatory molecules such as IL-1α, TNF-β, and GM-CSF. This is followed by the proliferation of antigen-specific cytotoxic CD8+ and also CD4+ (Th1) lymphocytes (Kimber I et al, 2002). These T lymphocytes disseminate via the efferent lymphatics throughout the body and interact with Langerhans' cells and residual antigen in the skin. When a sensitised person is re-exposed to the specific allergen, reaction between the allergen residues and the sensitised T-lymphocytes leads to elicitation of local reaction, termed as 'late' reaction.

Flow chart 3.1: Pathogenesis of allergic contact dermatitis

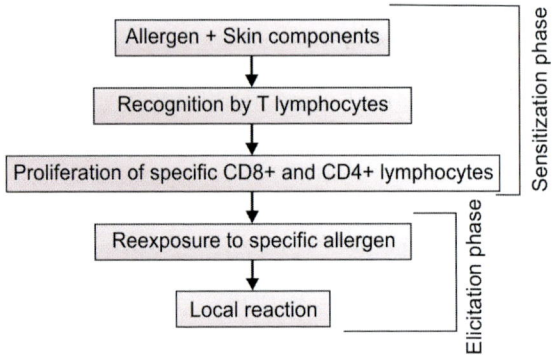

Predisposing Factors (Flow chart 3.2)

Flow chart 3.2: Predisposing factors of allergic contact dermatitis

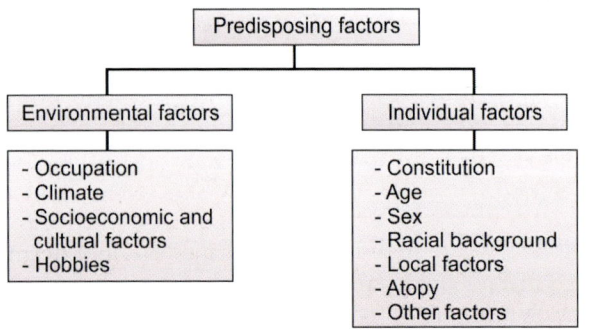

Individual Factors

1. *Constitution:* The capacity for sensitization varies individually, but some persons are more prone to develop sensitivity to a particular substance. Susceptibility to contact allergens may be a genetically determined trait (Menné T et al, 1986). On the contrary, studies on twins with hand eczema and nickel allergy indicate that environmental rather than genetic factors are important (Bryld LE et al, 2004).

2. *Age:* Age has a little influence on capacity for sensitization (Kwangsukstith C et al, 1995). The inflammatory response decreases with increasing age. But the number of positive patch-test reactions tends to increase with age (Berit CC et al, 2007), due to the accumulation of allergies. Young adults are more likely to have occupational or cosmetic allergies, whereas elderly people are more liable to medicament (Green CM et al, 2007) and 'historic' sensitivities.

3. *Sex:* Gender differences in the development of ACD are largely unknown. Female preponderance in clinical patch-test studies can be explained by exposure (Modjtahedi BS et al, 2004), for example, the large number of metal sensitive females, is a result of ear piercing (Peltonen L et al, 1989), and the greater exposure to fragrances, cosmetics and hair dyes.

4. *Racial background:* Some differences in prevalence of sensitization to individual allergens among racial groups have been observed, but this could be a reflection of exposure rather than predisposition (Deleo VA et al, 2002). Some reports implicate darker skin to have a heightened barrier function for a few substances thus lowering the respective risk for ACD (Reed JT et al, 1995).

5. *Local factors:* Pre-existing or concomitant constitutional and/or irritant contact dermatitis damages the skin, affecting its barrier function and increasing percutaneous absorption of allergens and secondary sensitization. Hand eczema predisposes to nickel sensitivity and *vice versa* (Menné T et al, 1982), and the prevalence of chromate, cobalt and balsam sensitivity is increased in men with hand eczema (Wilkinson DS et al, 1970). Occlusion greatly promotes percutaneous absorption and contributes to the high incidence of medicament dermatitis in stasis eczema, otitis externa and perianal dermatitis, and is also a factor in dermatitis from shoes and rubber gloves.

6. *Atopy:* The relationship of atopy, particularly atopic eczema, to predisposition to allergic contact dermatitis is not clear. Atopics exhibit down-regulation of Th1 cells, which should result in a decreased tendency to develop ACD. However, clinical studies are conflicting, some showing an increase in prevalence of contact allergy, especially to medicaments (Brandmann HJ et al, 1972), others the same (Cronin E et al, 1970) or a decrease (Hanifin JH, 1982).

7. *Other factors:* Hormones may have some effect on ACD. Contact dermatitis may flare premenstrually, with patch test reactivity to nickel being less intense during the ovulatory than the progestagenic phase (Bonamonte D et al, 2005). Drugs may also have an influence on ACD. Antihistamines have a little effect, whereas prednisolone (dose >15 mg/day), potent topical steroids (Moed H et al, 2004), immunosuppressants like azathioprine, cyclosporine, and UVB or psoralen UVA (PUVA) therapy suppress allergic patch-test reactions. Patients with acute or debilitating diseases like cancer, Hodgkin's disease and mycosis fungoides, have impaired capacity for contact sensitization (Grossman J et al, 1975).

Environmental Factors

1. *Occupation:* Occupational ACD is a common occurrence, and frequently complicates occupational irritant contact dermatitis. Individuals involved in carpet and footwear industry are exposed to various allergens like leather, formaldehyde, rubber, and dyeing agents.

2. *Climate:* Several factors like varying UV exposure, heat and relative humidity influence the seasonal liability to contact dermatitis. UVB exposure diminishes the skin's immune response to contact allergens. Seasonal variation of the dermatitic lesions may point towards a plant allergen or photo aggravation or photo allergy.

3. *Socioeconomic and cultural factors:* Exposure to cheap (nickel-releasing) metals used as jewellery is relatively higher in those with less disposable income. Similarly, the pattern of perfume and cosmetic exposure might vary according to social class. Cultural factors are also important, for example, hair dyes are used much more commonly by men in the Indian subcontinent, including use on the beard, Indian women may become

sensitized to dyes and adhesives used in kumkum and bindi applied to the forehead (Dwyer CM et al, 1994) (Fig. 3.1). The frequency of tattooing and body piercing has increased amongst young adults, thereby increasing their risk of contact with potential allergens including nickel and *p*-phenylenediamine (Fig. 3.2).

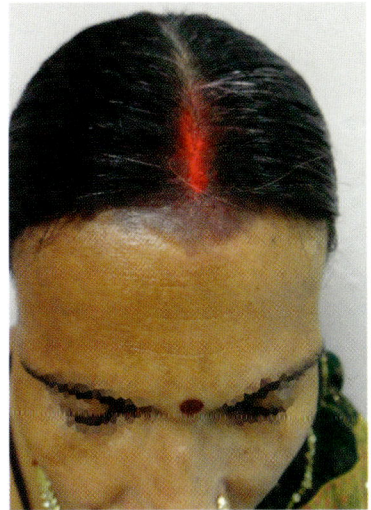

Fig. 3.1: ACD on forehead to sindoor (kumkum)

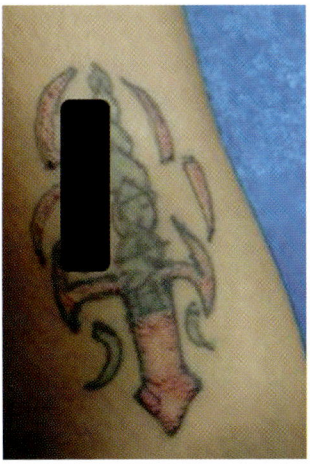

Fig. 3.2: Pruritic papules at the sites of red colored tattoo

4. *Hobbies:* Interests in gardening, cookery, painting, photography, etc. are considered important factors in causing ACD.

Clinical Features

The dominant symptom of ACD is itching. The classical clinical presentation of ACD is pruritic eczematous dermatitis. In early stages, it presents as erythema, swelling, papules and papulovesicles. Continued or repeated exposure to allergen might lead to dryness, thickening, and scaling of skin along with lichenification and fissuring in more chronic cases. ACD might occasionally present as non-eczematous reactions such as contact urticaria, erythema multiforme-like, purpuric, lichenoid, lymphomatoid, pigmented, leukoderma (Fig. 3.3), granulomatous, onycholysis and systematized contact dermatitis.

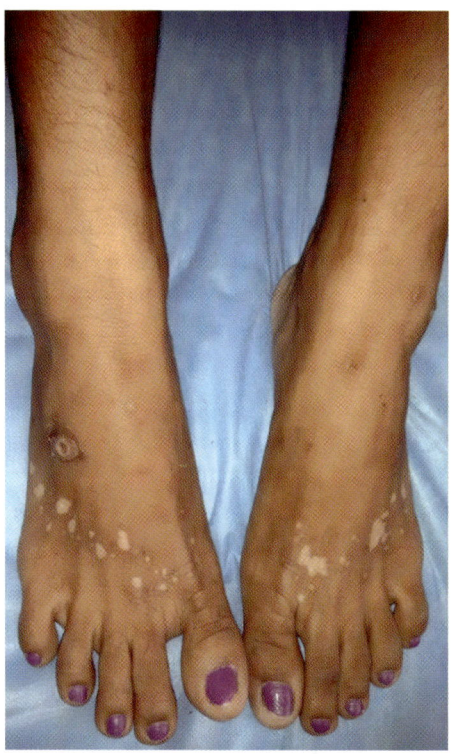

Fig. 3.3: Contact leukoderma due to footwear

History

The important points in history are summarised in Table 3.1.

Table 3.1: History taking in allergic contact dermatitis

Primary site	Important clue for diagnosis
Duration and behavior	Did the condition spread and if so where? Has the problem been persistent or intermittent? Are there any obvious exacerbating factors? Repeated sudden exacerbations may point to an ACD.
Previous history	Skin reactions to cheap metal, perfume and adhesive plasters, atopic diathesis (h/o infantile or childhood flexural eczema, asthma, hay fever or conjunctivitis)
Sources of allergy	i. Occupation, past and present: Improvement of dermatitis during weekends or holidays favors an occupational origin. ii. Hobbies (cement, glues, paint, wood and wood preservatives): Relapse at weekends suggests a hobby or non-occupational allergen. iii. Personal objects (textiles, footwear, protective clothing and gloves, jewellery, spectacles, hearing aids, medical appliances, cosmetics, toiletries, fragrances). iv. Home environment v. Current and previous topically applied medicaments: Dermatitis around a wound, especially leg ulcers, suggests sensitization to medicaments.
Medical history	Drug allergies, concomitant diseases, medications, surgeries.

Examination

The location can be important for identification of the causal allergen, since contact dermatitis is generally restricted to the contact site (Table 3.2).

Table 3.2: Common sources of ACD according to various sites

S. No.	Site	Common sources	Allergens
1.	Hands	Gloves, plants, cement	Latex, rubber, plant allergens, chromate
2.	Wrists	Watch, watchstraps	Nickel, chromate, colophony
3.	Forearms	Bracelets, bangles, dust, textiles, cement	Nickel, chromate, colophony, 4-phenylenediamine
4.	Face	Cosmetics, hair dyes, spectacle frames, preservatives, nail varnish, leather airband	Fragrances, Balsam of Peru, paraben, formaldehyde, 4-phenylenediamine, colo phony, nickel plastics, chromate
5.	Eyelids	Eye make-up, eye make-up removers and applicators, nail varnish, eye drops and ointments, contact lens solutions, plants	Fragrances, parabens, epoxy resins, colophony, Balsam of Peru, nickel, rubber, neomycin, gentamicin, preservatives plant allergens
6.	Lips and perioral area	Lipsticks, lip salves, medicaments, flavorings, garlic, cosmetics, toothpaste, chewing gum, dentures	Eosin, nickel, neomycin, gentamicin, paraben, preservatives, food additives, cinnamic aldehyde, spearmint oil, peppermint oil, colophony
7.	Ears	Earrings and clips, medicaments, hairpins, matches, hearing-aids, headsets, spectacle frame, nail varnish	Nickel, chromate, neomycin, plastics, epoxy resins, colophony, phosphorus sesquisulphide, urea, rubber
8.	Neck	Necklaces, zip-fasteners, nail varnish, textiles, perfumes	Nickel, chromate, epoxy resins, 4-phenylenediamine, fragrances
9.	Axilla	Deodrants, perfumes	Fragrances, Balsam of Peru
10.	Trunk	Clothes, buttons, zip-fasteners, elastic, leather belts, plants	Nickel, rubber, chromate, plant allergens
11.	Anogenital area	Medicaments, tights, toilet tissues and wipes, condoms	Neomycin, gentamicin, preservatives, local anesthetics, rubber
12.	Thighs	Textiles, coins	Nickel
13.	Lower legs	Medicaments, compression bandage, elastic hosiery	Topical antibiotics, rubber, colophony, nylon dye
14.	Feet	Shoes, stockings, topical medicaments, antiperspirants.	Rubber, colophony, nickel, preservatives
15.	Scalp	Hair dyes, hair styling products, medicated shampoos, minoxidil	4-phenylenediamine, preservatives, tar, zinc pyrithione

Hand dermatitis: About two-thirds of all cases of contact dermatitis involve the hands. The etiology is usually multifactorial, and includes both exogenous factors (exposure to irritants and allergens), and endogenous factors (atopy and defective skin barrier). Housewives' dermatitis, occupational dermatitis, and allergy to gloves are mostly confined to hands. Streaky dermatitis on the fingers, dorsa of the hands and forearms are typically caused by plants. Allergy to nickel, chromate and *p*-tertiary-butylphenol formaldehyde resin may develop at the wrists from sensitivity to the metal, leather and glue, respectively, in watchstraps containing these allergens. The forearms may be affected by the sensitizers that splash above protective gloves, particularly at work. Loose bracelets and bangles can also primarily involve forearms (Fig. 3.4).

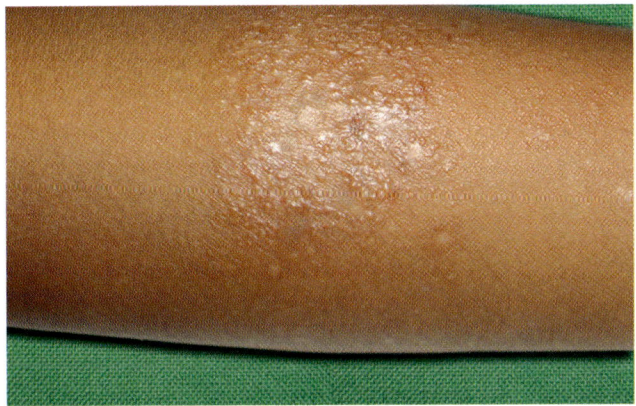

Fig. 3.4: ACD on forearms due to metal (Ni induced) bangles

FACE DERMATITIS

Facial allergic contact dermatitis from fragrances, hair dyes, preservatives and other constituents of skincare products and cosmetics, including nail varnish, is common. Nail varnish allergy often affects face in well-demarcated patches, and may be associated with eyelid dermatitis (Lidén C et al, 1993). A similar distribution may be seen from allergy to acrylic nails and rubber sponge applicators (Tucker SC et al, 1999). The forehead is affected by allergy to anything applied to the hair. Spectacle frames containing nickel or plastics may cause dermatitis on areas of contact with the cheeks, nose, eyelids and ears.

Eyelid dermatitis: The skin of the eyelids is thin, sensitive and may be sensitized by the fingers (e.g. nail varnish), airborne droplets (e.g. fragrance sprays) or volatile substances (e.g. epoxy resin). The common sources are eye creams, eye shadows, mascara, eye make-up removers, eyelash curlers and makeup applicators (nickel and/or rubber), eye drops and ointments, and contact lens solutions (preservatives).

Perioral dermatitis: ACD may occur from lipsticks and lip salves, nickel, medicaments, flavorings, garlic, and cosmetic excipients. Allergy to toothpaste (flavors), chewing gums (colophony), food additives (sodium metabisulphite), preservatives, colors, antioxidants, and badly fitting dentures are the potential causes of cheilitis and perioral eczema.

Ear lobe dermatitis: The ear, particularly the helix, may be sensitized by hair sprays, shampoos, and hair dyes. Earlobe dermatitis is a cardinal sign of nickel sensitivity in persons wearing artificial jewellery (Fig. 3.5). Ear piercing is often a precipitating factor in nickel and gold sensitivity. ACD can also be caused by

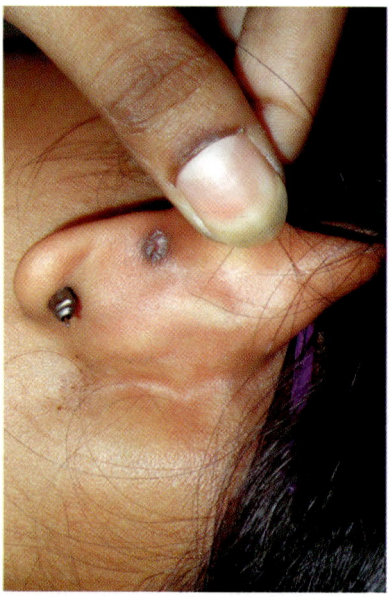

Fig. 3.5: ACD at the site of ear-piercing (nickel sensitivity)

habitual scratching with hairpins, pens or pencils (nickel), matches (phosphorus sesquisulphide and chromate) (Tucker SC et al, 1999) or fingertips (nail varnish), sensitizing medications (neomycin) (Fig. 3.6), clips (nickel), plastic helmets or bathing caps, spectacle frames (nickel and palladium), hearing aids, headsets, earphones, or earplugs.

Neck: ACD of neck can be caused by nickel in the clasps of necklaces or zip fasteners, nail varnish or primin from fingertips, perfume (sides of the neck), textiles (finishes in collars, dyes) and necklaces (nickel, exotic wood) which cause collar-like dermatitis, or eruptions on the sides of the neck. Dermatitis from airborne allergens and photosensitizers is sharply limited by the collar to the 'V' of the neck if blouses or open-necked shirts are worn.

Axilla: Allergic sensitivity may occur to fragrances in deodrants, and perfumes. The dermatitis produced by textiles tends to be periaxillary.

Trunk: Nickel buttons and zip fasteners may cause dermatitis localized to where they are worn, but a more widespread

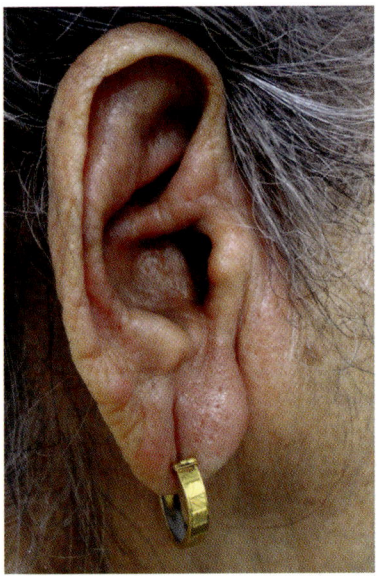

Fig. 3.6: Swelling and erythema as an allergic response to neomycin

secondary spread eruption is often associated. Chromate sensitivity from leather, and rubber allergy from elastic may present as truncal eczema (Fig. 3.7). Dermatitis from dresses, blouses and sweaters (textile dyes and finishes) usually predominantly affects the neck and folds of the axilla, and spares areas of skin covered by undergarments (Beck M H et al, 2010).

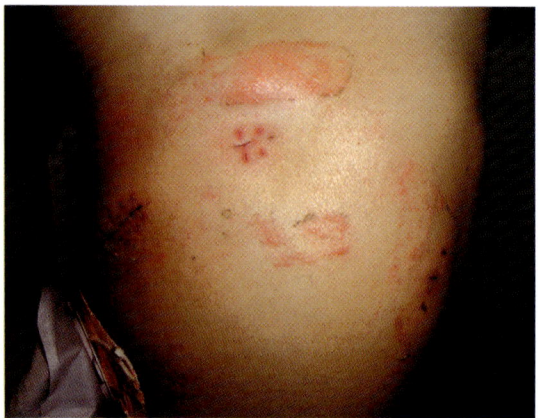

Fig. 3.7: ACD due to adhesive tape

Anogenital: The anogenital region is a common site for sensitization by medicaments for pruritus, skin eruptions and hemorrhoids (perfume, local anesthetics), neomycin, hydroxy-quinolines, ethylenediamine, corticosteroids, topical antifungals, moist toilet tissues and wipes (preservative), feminine hygiene sprays, condoms (rubber accelerators), nail varnish, tights (nylon dyes) (Beck M H et al, 2010).

Thighs: Textile dermatitis starts at the edge of the underwear, and is more pronounced in the popliteal spaces or gluteal folds. Finishes in the material of the pockets or objects kept in the pockets (e.g. nickel coins or boxes of matches) may produce a patch of dermatitis on the underlying skin as allergens may penetrate working clothes.

Lower legs: ACD from medicaments and dressings predominates, especially in those with varicose eczema and ulcers. The common medicament allergens are topical antibiotics and components of creams and paste bandages, such as lanolin, cetearyl alcohol and preservatives (Wilson CL et al, 1991). ACD can also be caused by compression bandaging (rubber, colophony) and elastic hosiery (rubber, nylon dye), rubber boots.

Foot: Dermatitis may result from shoe materials including leather, rubber, glues and nickel (Fig. 3.8), stockings, topical medicaments, antiseptics and antiperspirants. It presents as pruritic papular and oozy rash on dorsae of toes and feet, sparing the toe webs.

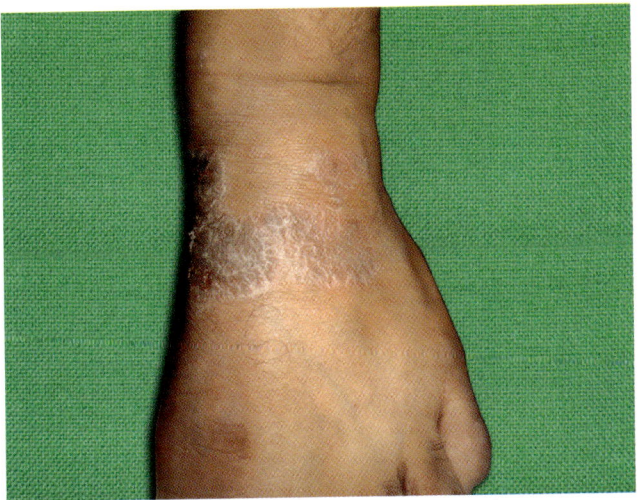

Fig. 3.8: Contact dermatitis due to footwear

Scalp: Scalp tends to be relatively spared from involvement by ACD. Dermatitis may still be caused by permanent hair dye, p-phenylenediamine, and related semi-permanent dyes (Fig. 3.9), hair-styling products such as mousses, gels, waxes and holding sprays, medicated shampoos (tar extract, zinc pyrithione, preservatives), and topical minoxidil (Friedman ES et al, 2002).

Generalized: Generalized erythroderma may be the result of a chronic contact dermatitis maintained by continued exposure to multiple allergens, including components of topical medicaments (Beck M H et al, 2010).

Systemically reactivated contact dermatitis: Ingestion or other systemic exposure to a contact allergen in an already sensitized

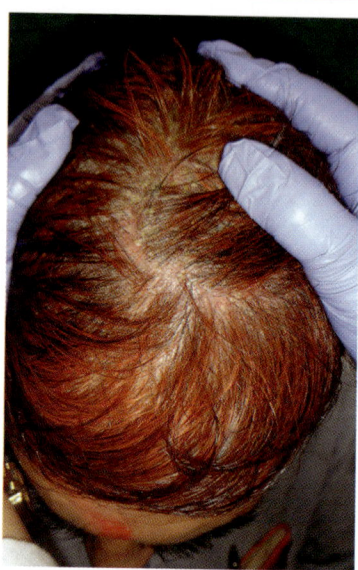

Fig. 3.9: Erythema and crusting on scalp (ACD to henna/mehendi)

person may result in a number of different patterns of skin eruption. Reactions may occur after systemic exposure to the primary allergen as well as closely related allergens. The most frequent types of reaction are focal flares of previous patch tests and sites of previous dermatitis, vesicular hand eczema, or more widespread eczema and erythema, sometimes with additional urticarial features.

Photoallergic contact dermatitis: Certain substances are transformed into irritants or sensitizers (photosensitizers) after irradiation with UV or short-wave visible radiation (280–600 nm). Photoallergic dermatitis is usually localized to exposed areas of the skin (Fig. 3.10), with well-demarcated margins where the skin is covered by clothing, for example, at the collar and 'V' of the neck, below the end of the sleeves and trouser leggings. The area below the chin and 'Wilkinson's triangle' behind the earlobe is usually spared (Wilkinson DS, 1962). The common photoallergens are UV filters, including p-aminobenzoic acid and its derivatives, cinnamates, benzophenones, perfumes (musk ambrette), halogenated salicylanilides used as antibacterials in soaps and detergents, topical non-steroidal anti-inflammatory agents like

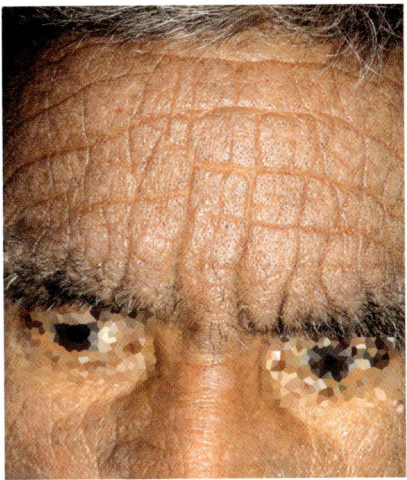

Fig. 3.10: Involvement of face in photoallergic contact dermatitis

ketoprofen, phenothiazines, topical sulphonamides, eosin in lipsticks, thiourea (in design paper), and garlic.

Diagnosis

Patch testing is the universally accepted method for the detection of causative contact allergens. A proper patch test uses a specific purified etiologic agent reproducing the clinical disease in a susceptible host and causing no disease outside the proper clinical settings (Fig. 3.11). To perform this test, specific allergens are applied on the upper back in Finn chambers (occlusive aluminum

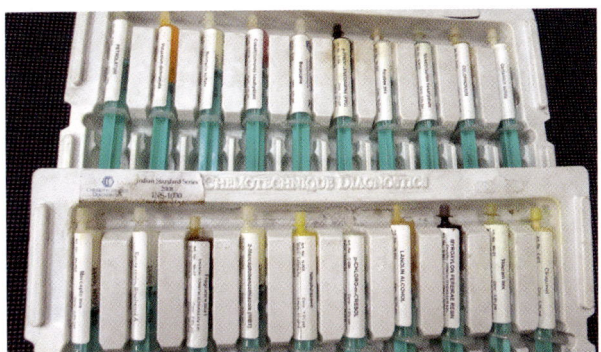

Fig. 3.11: Battery of allergens in Indian standard series patch test kit

discs) under occlusion. Standard series include those allergens which most commonly cause reactions in the population, and to detect other less common ones which may not be considered by history or distribution of dermatitis being investigated. The allergens in Indian standard series are listed in Table 3.3.

Table 3.3: Allergens in Indian standard series and their common sources

S. No.	Compound	conc. % (W/W)	Vehicle	Common sources
1.	Petrolatum white (pet)	100.0	Pet	Base/vehicle
2.	Potassium dichromate	0.5	Pet	Cement, antirust paints, dust liberated by drilling, cutting or sandpapering of painted metals
3.	Neomycin sulfate	20.0	Pet	Topical antibiotic, cross reaction with kanamycin, framycetin (soframycin), gentamicin, tobramycin
4.	Cobalt chloride hexahydrate	1.0	Pet	Hard metal used for metal cutting and drilling, magnets, jewellery, alloys, paints, glass, china pottery, ceramics
5.	Benzocaine	5.0	Pet	Local anesthetic
6.	4-phenylenediamine base	1.0	Pet	Hair dyes, tattoos, henna, textile azo dyes
7.	Paraben mix	15.0	Pet	Preservative in topical and parenteral medicaments, paste bandages, cosmetics, ultrasound gels and foods.
8.	Nickel sulphate hexahydrate	5.0	Pet	Alloys, plated objects, jewellery and metal components of clothing, coins, keys, scissors, knitting needles, other metallic tools, utensils, diet.
9.	Colophony	20.0	Pet	Pine trees and wood, adhesive dressings, glues, balms and salves, printing ink, herbal medicaments
10.	Gentamicin	20.0	Pet	Topical antibiotic
11.	Epoxy resins	1.0	Pet	Coatings including paints, varnishes and metals, construction industry, dental fillings, cardiac pacemakers

Contd.

Table 3.3: Allergens in Indian standard series and their common sources
(Contd.)

S. No.	Compound	conc. % (W/W)	Vehicle	Common sources
12.	Fragrance mix	8.0	Pet	Perfumes, cosmetics, moisturizers, deodorants, aftershaves, soaps, bath additives, aromatherapy oils, toilet tissues and wipes
13.	2-mercapto-benzothiazole	2.0	Pet	Rubber industry, rubber gloves, shoes, gloves, clothing, condoms, electric cords, tubes, masks, rubber bands
14.	Nitrofurazone	1.0	Pet	Topical antibiotic
15.	Chlorocresol	1.0	Pet	Corticosteroid creams, topical medicaments
16.	Wool alcohols	30.0	Pet	Cosmetics (creams, lotions, ointments), topical drugs
17.	Balsam of Peru	25.0	Pet	Perfumes, cosmetics, medicaments, e.g. hemorrhoid preparations, balms for wounds, sprains, joint pains, flavor in tobacco, spices, drinks
18.	Thiuram mix	1.0	Pet	Rubber industry, rubber gloves, shoes, gloves, clothing, condoms, electric cords, tubes, masks, rubber bands
19.	Clioquinol	5.0	Pet	Topical medicaments
20.	Black rubber mix	0.6	Pet	Rubber industry, rubber gloves, shoes, gloves, clothing, condoms, electric cords, tubes, masks, rubber bands
21.	4-tert-butyl-phenolformaldehyde resin	1.0	Pet	Electrical appliances, glues, plywood, fiberglass, brake linings, telephones and steering wheels
22.	Formaldehyde	1.0	Aqueous (aq)	Cosmetics, clothing resins, shampoos, paints/lacquers, glues, printing ink, used for preservation of pathological specimens, orthopedic casts, renal dialysis
23.	Polyethyleneglycol	100.0	Aqueous (aq)	Cosmetics (shampoos, hair dressings), topical medicaments, detergents
24.	Parthenolide	0.1	Pet	Herbal medicaments

Readings are made after 2 and 4 days, one hour after removal of patch tests. The patch test reactions are recorded as follows (International Contact Dermatitis Research Group) (Wilkinson DS et al, 1970):

-    Negative
- ?+   Doubtful reaction; faint erythema only
- +   Weak positive reaction; palpable erythema, infiltration, possibly papules
- ++   Strong positive reaction; erythema, infiltration, papules, vesicles
- +++ Extreme positive reaction; intense erythema and infiltration and coalescing vesicles
- IR   Irritant reaction of different types
- NT Not tested

Reading at day 4 is important to distinguish an allergic from a false-positive non-allergic irritant reaction. No infiltration, lack of itching, deep redness or a brown hue, and sharp delineation corresponding to the margins of the patch test point to an irritant reaction. It is important to rule out false positive and false negative reactions.

A positive reaction confirms the person has allergic contact sensitivity, although this does not necessarily mean that the substance is the cause of the presenting clinical dermatitis, and it is important to establish relevance by carefully re-examining the patient's history, distribution of rash and materials with which there has been contact.

The adverse patch test reactions include active sensitization, folliculitis, irritant reactions, ectopic flare of dermatitis, Koebner's phenomenon, hyper or hypopigmentation at test sites, scarring, and anaphylaxis (rare).

Other adjunctive tests for diagnosis of ACD include open test, TRUE test, repeat open application test, Usage test, and intradermal test. Photoallergic contact dermatitis is diagnosed by photopatch testing.

Differential Diagnosis

Allergic contact dermatitis should be differentiated from irritant contact dermatitis, atopic dermatitis, asteatotic dermatitis, dyshidrotic eczema, nummular dermatitis, autosensitization reaction, mycosis fungoides, stasis dermatitis, psoriasis, and seborrheic dermatitis.

Prevention

Principles of prevention can be divided into primary, secondary and tertiary. Primary prevention focuses on the induction of contact sensitization and control of exposure. Secondary prevention relates to elicitation, and tertiary to measures for established and continuing dermatitis. Containment, replacement and elimination of potential allergenic hazards can be helpful in both the domestic and working environments, for example, perfume-free cosmetics and medicaments, non-latex gloves, high molecular-weight epoxy resins (Thorgeirsson A et al, 1978), and white spirit instead of turpentine. Housewives' dermatitis can be prevented by wearing cotton-lined gloves when the hands are in contact with irritants, including food, cleaning agents and polishes. Skin protection courses and education have been shown to reduce occupational dermatitis.

Treatment

The first principle of management is to give advice on avoidance of the possible sources of sensitizer and cross-reacting substances. Examples of specific avoidance measures include plastic instead of rubber gloves, cosmetics and medicaments free of an identified allergen, and clothing free of nickel-containing studs, zips, etc. It should be stressed that allergy does not disappear when the dermatitis clears but that the risk of relapse after further contact with the allergen persists throughout life.

Topical steroids are used in the acute stage and are gradually replaced by hydrating emollients as the skin lesions improve. It is important to choose the topical corticosteroid to which the patient is not allergic. Topical calcineurin inhibitors should be considered when steroid-sparing agents are required, and for certain areas like face, axilla, groins where chances of steroid-induced atrophy are high. In severe and widespread cases, systemic corticosteroids may be indicated for a short period of time. Secondary infection requires antibiotics, and a sedative antihistamine is indicated for pruritus, particularly at night. Recalcitrant, disabling cases may require treatment with immunosuppressive therapy such as azathioprine (Verma KK et al, 2000) and ciclosporin.

Prognosis

The prognosis of ACD depends on its cause and the feasibility of avoiding repeated or continued exposure to the causative allergen. Associated irritant dermatitis and constitutional factors are also important. Prognosis of ACD is worse than irritant contact dermatitis. It is clear from a number of studies that poor compliance and understanding results in a higher rate of ongoing exposure to the causative allergen, and is associated with a worse prognosis (Agner T et al, 1999). Once relevant allergens are identified by patch test and successfully avoided, improvement of dermatitis is the rule.

Sensitivity to ubiquitous allergens, such as nickel and chromate (Thormann J et al, 1979), and to strong allergens, such as primin and PPD (Fisher AA et al, 1958), is reported to persist, whereas sensitivity to other weaker and avoidable allergens may disappear.

Bibliography

1. Adams RM. Diagnostic patch testing. In: Occupational Skin Disease. New York: Grune and Stratton 1983: 136.

2. Agner T, Flyvholm MA, Menné T. Formaldehyde allergy: a follow-up study. Am J Contact Dermatitis 1999; 10: 12–7.

3. Ayto J. Dictionary of Word Origins. London: Bloomsbury 1990: 18.

4. Bandmann H-J, Breit R, Leutgeb C. Kontakallergie und Dermatitis atopica. Arch Dermatol Forsch 1972;244: 332–4.

5. Beck M. H, Wilkinson B.M. Allergic contact dermatitis. In: burns T, Breathnach SM, Cox N, Griffiths C, editors. Rook's Textbook of Dermatology. 8th Ed. Oxford. Blackwell; 2010: 26.1–106.

6. Berit CC, Menné T, Johansen JD. 20 years of standard patch testing in an eczema population with focus on patients with multiple contact allergies. Contact Dermatitis 2007;57: 76–83.

7. Bonamonte D, Foti C, Antelmi AR, Biscozzi AM et al. Nickel contact allergy and menstrual cycle. Contact Dermatitis 2005;52: 309–13.

8. Bryld LE, Hindsberger C, Kyvik KO et al. Genetic factors in nickel allergy evaluated in a population-based female twin sample. J Invest Dermatol 2004;123: 1025–9.

9. Cronin E, Bandmann H-J, Calnan CD et al. Contact dermatitis in the atopic. Acta Derm Venereol (Stockh) 1970; 50: 183–7.

10. Deleo VA, Taylor SC, Belsito DV et al. The effect of race and ethnicity on patch test results. J Am Acad Dermatol 2002;46: S107–12.

11. Dwyer CM, Forsyth A. Allergic contact dermatitis from bindi. Contact Dermatitis 1994;30: 174.

12. Fisher AA, Prelzig A, Kanof NB. The persistence of allergic eczematous sensitivity and the cross-sensitivity pattern to paraphenylenediamine. J Invest Dermatol 1958; 30: 9–12.

13. Friedman ES, Friedman PM, Cohen DE et al. Allergic contact dermatitis to topical minoxidil solution: etiology and treatment. J Am Acad Dermatol 2002;46: 309–12.

14. Green CM, Holden CR, Gawkrodger DJ. Contact allergy to topical medicaments becomes more common with advancing age: an age-stratifi ed study. Contact Dermatitis 2007;56: 229–31.

15. Grossman J, Baum J, Gluckman J et al. The effect of aging and acute illness on delayed hypersensitivity. J Allergy Clin Immunol 1975;55: 262–75.

16. Hanifin JH. Atopic dermatitis. J Am Acad Dermatol 1982;6: 1–13.

17. Heine G, Schnuch A, Uter W, Worm M. Frequency of contact allergy in German children and adolescents patch tested between 1995 and 2002: results from the Information Network of Departments of Dermatology and the German Contact Dermatitis Research Group. Contact Dermatitis 2004; 51: 111–7.

18. Kimber I, Dearman RJ. Allergic contact dermatitis: the cellular effects. Contact Dermatitis 2002;46: 1–5.

19. Kwangsukstith C, Maibach HI. Effects of age and sex on the induction and elicitation of allergic contact dermatitis. Contact Dermatitis 1995;33: 289–98.

20. Lepoittevin J-P. Molecular aspects of allergic contact dermatitis. In: Frosch PJ, Menné T, Lepoittevin J-P, eds. Contact Dermatitis, 4th edn. Berlin: Springer, 2006: 45–68.

21. Lidén C, Berg M, Farm G et al. Nail varnish allergy with far-reaching consequences. Br J Dermatol 1993;128: 57–62.

22. Menné T, Borgan O, Green A. Nickel allergy and hand dermatitis in a stratified sample of the Danish female population. Acta Derm Venereol (Stockh) 1982;62: 35–41.

23. Menné T, Holm V. Genetic susceptibility in human allergic sensitization. Semin Dermatol 1986;5: 301–6.

24. Modjtahedi BS, Modjtahedi SP, Maibach HI. The sex of the individual as a factor in allergic contact dermatitis. Contact Dermatitis 2004;50: 53–9.

25. Moed H, Stoof TJ, Boorsma DM et al. Identification of anti-inflammatory drugs according to their capacity to suppress type-1 and type-2 T cell profiles. Clin Exp Allergy 2004; 34: 1868–75.

26. Peltonen L, Terho P. Nickel sensitivity in schoolchildren in Finland. In: Frosch P, Dooms-Goossens A, LaChapelle J-M et al., eds. Current Topics in Contact Dermatitis. Heidelberg: Springer, 1989: 184–7.

27. Reed JT, Ghadially R, Elias PM. Skin type, but neither race nor gender, influence epidermal permeability barrier function. Arch Dermatol 1995;33: 289–98.

28. Sharma VK, Asati DP. Pediatric contact dermatitis. Indian J Dermatol Venereol Leprol 2010;76: 514–20.

29. Thorgeirsson A, Fregert S, Fammas O. Sensitization capacity of epoxy resin oligomers in the guinea pig. Acta Derm Venereol (Stockh) 1978; 58: 17–21.

30. Thormann J, Jesperson NB, Joensen HD. Persistence of contact allergy to chromium. Contact Dermatitis 1979; 5: 261–5.

31. Tucker SC, Beck MH. A 15-year study of patch testing to (meth) acrylates. Contact Dermatitis 1999;40: 278–9.

32. Tucker SC, Lyon CC, Beck MH. Persistent otitis externa due to allergic contact dermatitis to phosphorus sesquisulphide in 'strike-anywhere' matches (Minerva). BMJ 1999; 318: 1566.

33. Verma KK, Manchanda Y, Pasricha JS. Azathioprine as a corticosteroid sparing agent for the treatment of dermatitis caused by the weed Parthenium. Acta Derm Venereol (Stockh) 2000; 80:31–2.

34. Wilkinson DS. Patch test reactions to certain halogenated salicylanilides. Br J Dermatol 1962;74: 302–6.

35. Wilkinson DS, Bandmann H-J, Calnan CD et al. The role of contact allergy in hand eczema. Trans St John's Hosp Dermatol Soc 1970;56: 15–9.

36. Wilkinson DS, Fregert S, Magnusson B et al. Terminology of contact dermatitis. Acta Derm Venereol (Stockh) 1970; 50: 287–92.

37. Wilson CL, Cameron J, Powell SM et al. High incidence of contact dermatitis in leg-ulcer patients: implications for management. Clin Exp Dermatol 1991;16: 25–03.

4

Non-Eczematous Contact Dermatitis

Besides the classic eczematous form of contact dermatitis (CD) detailed in the previous chapter (Chapter 3) a number of non-eczematous clinical variants have also been described, which are often misdiagnosed, a few of which are being detailed below.

1. Erythema Multiforme-like Contact Dermatitis

Of all the types this is believed to be the most common type in the West and is commonly due to exotic woods, medicaments, and ethylenediamine.

Clinical Features

Early lesions are eczematous and localized at the allergen contact site. After 1 to 15 days delay, the erythema multiforme-like eruption follows, involving the area around the original lesions or extending to the whole cutaneous surface. The generalized spread is due to systemic exposition to drugs which the patient had previously been sensitized to topically.

Target-like, erythematovesicular, or urticarial lesions are characteristic. Resolution is slow-paced; these manifestations persist usually much longer than the original eczematous lesions (or sometimes appearing after regression of the latter).

2. Purpuric Contact Dermatitis (PCD)

This particular form of noneczematous contact dermatitis is frequently misdiagnosed. The eruption evolves in several weeks after the withdrawal of the offending agent and resolves with more or less persistent pigmentation. It can be secondary to irritant, or more frequently allergic, mechanisms.

Causes

a. *Rubber:* This has been associated with the use of rubber boots, rubber diving suits, elasticized shorts, and rubberized support leg bandage. It has also been seen due to the use of orthopedic elastic bandages.

b. *Textile:* This was initially associated with optical whiteners, but has been described due to various dyes added to clothing. A petechial and itchy dermatitis is seen in those areas which are typically subject to tighter contact with clothes (*armpits, arms, upper limbs folds, neck and thighs*).

Clinical Features

Purpuric contact dermatitis can be either toxic or allergic in nature. Palpable purpuric lesions are seen followed by persistent pigmentation. At times, clinical extension represents a useful feature in differentiating the 2 forms, the irritant being strictly limited to contact sites.

3. Lichenoid Contact Dermatitis

A particularly uncommon form of noneczematous contact dermatitis which presents with clinical features resembling those of lichen planus. It affects both skin and mucosal membranes.

Causes: Color developers, substances derived from paraphenylenediamine, are the most common cause of allergic contact lichenoid eruption. As a general rule, the eruption from color developers spares the oral mucosa. Cases from paraphenylenediamine in hair dyes, *P. obconica*, nickel, epoxy resins, aminoglycoside antibiotics and methacrylic acid esters for industrial use have been reported. Oral mucosae can be involved due to copper, zinc, and mercury contained in dental restorations.

Clinical Features

Eczematous lesions evolve into lichenoid papular lesions. Though the eruption mostly involves contact sites, it can spread widely but usually spares the mucosa. The course is prolonged and leaves variably intense pigmentary changes lasting up to some months.

4. Pigmented Contact Dermatitis/Riehl's Melanosis

One of the reason that this is being covered here is that this condition is often misdiagnosed as lichen planus pigmentosis or ashy dermatoses and the patient is put on various topical and systemic agents which rarely help, complicating the condition as the irritation caused by the topical agents aggravate the condition. As this is caused commonly by cosmetics, which is a largely unregulated industry, it is this author's belief that a large number of such cases are missed in clinical practice!

Pigmented contact dermatitis was first reported by Osmundsen in Denmark in 1969. In 8 months he had 120 patients, seven of whom showed a pronounced and bizarre hyperpigmentation. In four of these seven cases, contact dermatitis preceded the hyperpigmentation, while the other three did not notice any signs of dermatitis, such as itching or erythema, before the pigmentation appeared.

Clinical Features

Hyperpigmentation, with or without dermatitis, was located mostly in *covered areas*, such as the chest, back, waist, arms, neck, and thighs. The hyperpigmentation was brown, slate-colored, grayish brown, reddish-brown, bluish-brown, etc. according to the case, and often had a reticulate pattern.

The cause was linked to the use of washing powders that contained a new optical whitener, Tinopal or CH3566. This was one of numerous optical whiteners that became available at that time to make textiles "whiter than white." Another cause was azo dyes and affected workers in a textile factory.

Prevention and Treatment

The problem in preventing lies in a knowledge of the countless chemicals that are used even now in the textile industry. The purity of dyes is, in general, very low and some of the many impurities are allergenic. The experiences accumulated in the past show that when entirely new textile finishes are introduced to the textile industry, the minimum safety evaluation tests such as *LD50, Ames test, and skin irritation test* should be performed, and their sensitization potential should be investigated by a research team including dermatologists.

Pigmented Cosmetic Dermatitis

The signs of pigmented cosmetic dermatitis are diffuse or reticular, black or dark-brown hyperpigmentation of the face, which cannot be cured by the use of corticosteroid ointments or the continuous ingestion of vitamin C.

Japanese dermatologists gradually became aware of the role of cosmetics in this hyperpigmentation. First, it occurred only in those women, and very exceptionally men, who used cosmetics, and secondly, even though the bizarre brown hyperpigmentation was so conspicuous, the presence of slight, recurrent, or preceding dermatitis was observed in most cases clinically or on taking a history.

Clinical Features

The border of pigmented cosmetic dermatitis is not sharp, as in lichen planus or melasma (Fig. 4.1). In some cases, the dark brown or black hyperpigmentation is also seen on skin other than on the face (Fig. 4.2). The neck (Figs 4.2 and 4.3), chest, and back can be involved and, in a few exceptional cases, hyperpigmentation may extend to the whole body. In these cases, the allergens cinnamic alcohol and its derivatives sensitize the patients first to cosmetics and then provoke allergic reactions to soaps, domestic fabric softeners, and food, all of which sometimes contain cinnamic derivatives.

Causative agents: Jasmine absolute, ylang-ylang oil, cananga oil, benzyl salicylate, hydroxycitronellal, sandalwood oil, artificial

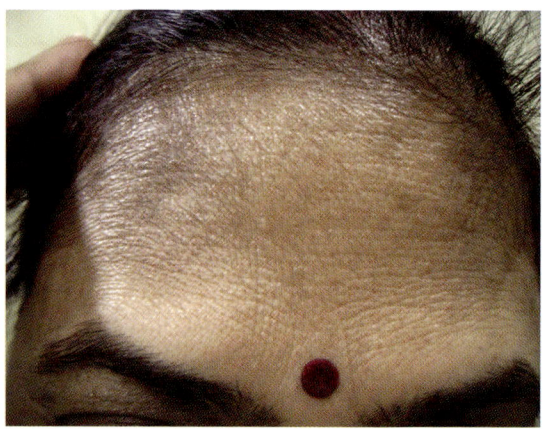

Fig. 4.1: A case of PCD (pigmented cosmetic dermatitis) on the forehead in a patient who was allergic to PPD and had been using hair dyes for more than 7 years

sandalwood, geraniol, geranium oil, D and C Red 31, Yellow No. 11 and PPD (Fig. 4.1). Other rare causations of pigmented cosmetic dermatitis include fragrances (Fig. 4.3), musk ambrette, musk moskene, pigment Orange F2G, and diisostearyl malate in the lipsticks.

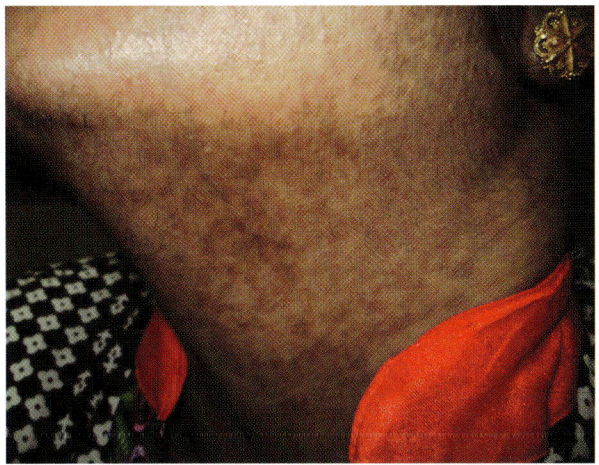

Fig. 4.2: A female with PCD extending to the neck, diagnosed as a case of lichen planus pigmentosus

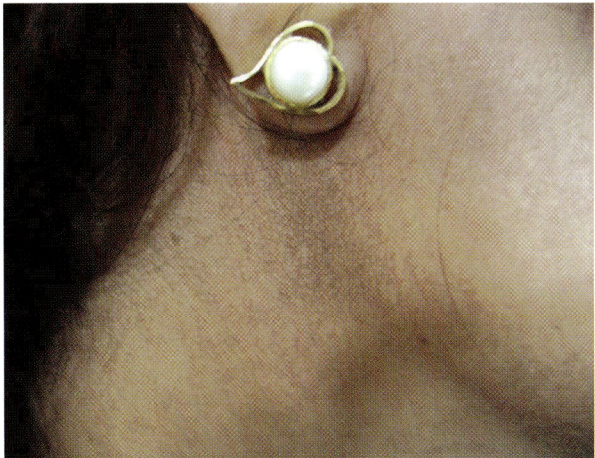

Fig. 4.3: An early case of PCD in a female using a fragrance on the jawline "pulse point"

Treatment

Stopping all kinds of facial creams, specially fairness creams and avoiding facials, perfumes, foundations and sunscreens are a tough protocol to follow, but I have seen patients with near complete improvement with such a protocol. This is as most of the causative allergens are difficult to find and thus its best to stop whatever is possible. It usually required **1–2 years** for a patient to regain normal nonhyperpigmented facial skin. The dermatologist may choose to administer a topical product with a long history of safety, but using a triple combination creams or a skin lightening cream is of little use.

In most cases contamination with ordinary soaps and cosmetics is a decisive factor inhibiting therapeutic results, because such ordinary daily necessities contain the allergens that cause the condition. Thus, it is a good advise to ask the patient to visit the dermatologist once a month to be checked for improvement where the patient is persuaded every time to avoid products used in beauty parlors.

Though not a definitive list Table 4.1 elucidates the common allergens that can cause this dermatoses.

Table 4.1: A list of agents that can cause pigmented contact and cosmetic dermatitis*

Optical whiteners	Tinopal CH 3566
Dyes	Naphthol AS Sudan I Brilliant lake red Vacanceine RedSolvent orange 8
Cosmetics	Pigments: Pigment orange 3 Pigment red 3 Pigment red 49 Pigment red 53 Pigment red 64 Azoic solvents: • Solvent orange 2 • Solvent orange 8
Fragrances	Cananga Geraniol

Contd.

Table 4.1: A list of agents that can cause pigmented contact and cosmetic dermatitis* (Contd.)

Optical whiteners	Tinopal CH 3566
Fragrances	Hydroxycitronellal
	Jasmine
	Patchouli
	Sandalwood oil
	Ylang-ylang
Miscellaneous agents	Formaldehyde
	Nickel
	Rubber
	Primula obconica
	Musk ambrette
	Cinnamic alcohol
	Benzyl salicylate
Lightening creams	Kojic acid
Hair dye	PPD

* Hideo Nakayama. Pigmented Contact Dermatitis and Chemical Depigmentation. J.D. Juhansen et al. (eds.): Contact Dermatitis, DOI: 10.1007/978-3-642-03827-3_19, © Springer-Verlag Berlin Heidelberg 2011.

5. Lymphomatoid Contact Dermatitis

This uncommon dermatitis manifests with the clinical features of plaque parapsoriasis or an early stage mycosis fungoides. The most frequent antigens are paraphenylenediamine, para-tertiary butylphenol resin, gold, ethylenediamine, and nickel. Lymphomatoid contact dermatitis and mycosis fungoides alike present with infiltrative patches; the former, however, demonstrates a bright erythematous color and undefined margins.

6. Pustular Contact Dermatitis

Pustules are usually associated with irritant reactions. Nevertheless, allergic pustular reactions are known from nitrofurazone, black rubber and minoxidil.

Bibliography

1. C.L. Goh, "Non-eczematous contact reactions," in Textbook of Contact Dermatitis, R.J.G. Rycroft, T. Menn'e, P.J. Frosh, and J.P. Lepoittevin, Eds., pp. 413–431, Springer, Berlin, Germany, 3rd edition, 2001.

2. Hideo Nakayama. Pigmented Contact Dermatitis and Chemical Depigmentation. J.D. Johansen et al. (eds.), Contact Dermatitis, DOI: 10.1007/978-3-642-03827-3_19, © Springer-Verlag Berlin Heidelberg 2011.

3. R. L. Rietschel and J. F. Fowler, "Noneczematous contact dermatitis," in Fisher's Contact Dermatitis 6. Hamilton, R.L. Rietschel and J. F. Fowler, Eds., pp. 88–109, BC Decker, 2008.

5

Photoallergic Eczema

PHOTOALLERGIC ECZEMA

Photoallergic reactions are usually triggered by sunlight and can persist in a chronic state as seen in chronic actinic dermatitis. The rash is seen on the areas exposed to the sun, its exact location is dictated by the clothes worn by the patient (Fig. 5.1). Generally speaking, it will be confined to the face, exposed area of the neck, nape of the neck, dorsum of the hands and the forearms (Fig. 5.2). It is a delayed type 4 hypersensitivity reaction.

In cases of contact photosensitization, the rash is confined to the areas to which the photoallergen has been applied. Thus, a photoallergic reaction to a daily care cream will occur only on the face (Fig. 5.3), a reaction to a topical anti-inflammatory agent will cause a rash on the treated joint; with phytophotodermatosis, only

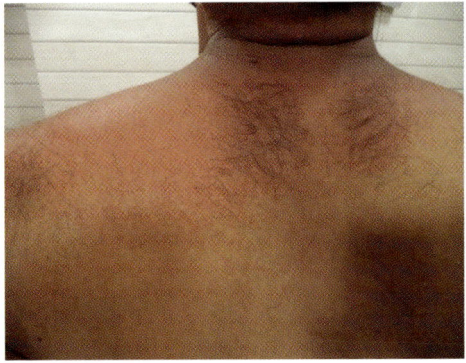

Fig. 5.1: A patient with an acute phototoxic reaction involving the upper back following exposure to sunlight while on a beach holiday

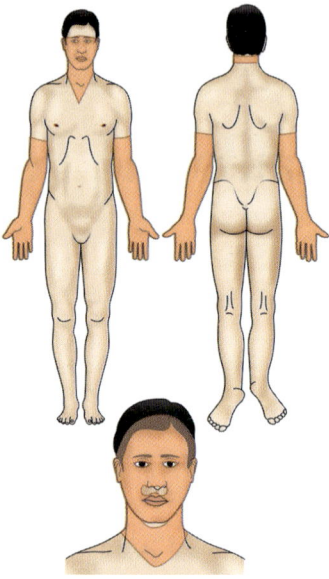

Fig. 5.2: A depiction of the distribution of a photoinduced reaction, which involves the exposed sites but spares the submental, supraorbital and periorbital area

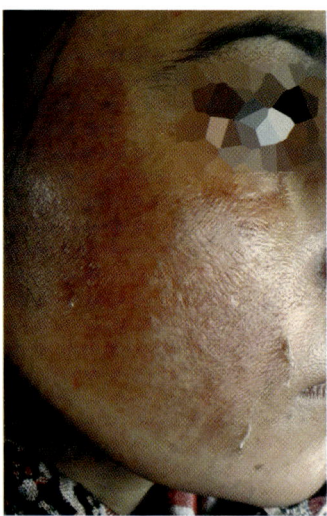

Fig. 5.3: An intense photoallergic reaction in a patient who used a herbal face pack. The peeling noticed is due to the use of topical corticosteroids that abates the intense erythema

the areas directly in contact with the plant will present the typical vesicular-bullous lesions.

In the event of systemic photosensitization, the photoallergen spreads evenly throughout the skin in such a way that all sun-exposed areas are affected simultaneously with only slight variations in intensity due to the impact of the sun's rays.

Types of Rash

The appearance of the rash varies depending on the patho-physiological mechanisms underlying the photosensitivity reaction.

Phototoxicity: A phototoxic reaction causes intense erythema (Fig. 5.1) sometimes with blistering and peeling resembling a sunburn. Once the rash heals, a marked post-inflammatory pigmentation is seen.

Photoallergy is a photoimmunologic reaction which, like contact dermatitis, involves the patient's immune system. It presents as eczema-like, lichenoid, or urticaria-like lesions. To begin with, the lesions are confined to sun-exposed areas but may spread to protected zones if the patient does not avoid the sun completely.

Etiology

In cases of *contact photosensitization*, the culpable substance is identified by carefully interviewing the patient to establish a list of all the topical agents, cosmetics (Fig. 5.3) and plants with which he or she has come into contact. Though a photopatch is frequently used, it must be borne in mind that any phototoxic substance will induce a positive photopatch-test result if sufficiently UV-irradiated. This means that an allergen cannot be identified on the basis of a positive photopatch-test result alone.

It is much more difficult to identify the responsible substance in cases of *systemic photosensitization*. All the medication taken by the patient, together with the doses taken and the dates started, must be noted down. Usually days started 3 to 14 days before the rash is the usual culprit (Table 5.1).

Investigation

Currently, the most effective and widely used method for investigating in a patient is to perform photopatch testing. In this process, agents under investigation are prepared in a vehicle (often

Table 5.1: The list of medicines with known photosensitizing potential

Antibacterials	Azithromycin
	Ciprofloxacin
	Doxycyclin
	Isoniazide
	Levofloxacin
	Lymecycline
	Minocycline
	Norfloxacin
	Ofloxacin
	Antifungal agents griseo-fulvin, itraconazole
	Voriconazole
Antimalarial agents	
Antiviral agents	Efavirenz ribavirin
Antidiabetic agents	Glibenclamide
	Glimepiride
	Glipizide
Anti-inflammatories	Diclofenac
	Ibuprofen
	Indomethacin
	Ketoprofen
	Naproxen
	Olsalazine
	Piroxicam
	Sulfasalazine
Antineoplastic agents	Methotrexate
	Imatinib
	Fluorouracil
Proton pump inhibitors	
Antihypertensive agents,	Captopril
anti-arrhythmic agents	Diltiazem
	Enalapril
	Nifedipine
	Ramipril
Diuretics	
Lipid-lowering agents	
Neuroleptics,	Amitriptyline
antidepressants	Carbamazepine

Contd.

Table 5.1: The list of medicines with known photosensitizing potential (Contd.)

	Chlorpromazine
	Fluoxetine
	Imipramine
	Levomepromazine
	Paroxetine
Topical drugs	Diclofenac
	Diphenhydramine
	Fluorouracil
	Benzole peroxide
Antiseptics	Bithionol
	Fentichlor
	Triclosan
Cosmetics	Para-aminobenzoic acid, cinnamates, octocrylene, benzophenones, dibenzoylmethane, benzylidene camphor (sun filters)
	Peru Balsam
	Eosin
	Bergamot essence
	Oak moss, 6-methylcoumarine (fragrances)
	Paraphenylenediamine (hair dyes)
Botanics	Furocoumarins (angelica, celery, lemon, fig, parsnip, parsley)
	Sesquiterpinic lactones (artichoke, chrysanthemum, dahlia, frullania, lettuce, lichen, dandelion)

petrolatum) and a small volume is placed within plastic or metal chambers, which have low chemical reactivity and are mounted on hypoallergenic adhesive tape. After the chamber preparation, they are then applied in duplicate sets to the skin of the patients' back. Ideally, the tape and chambers should not be placed on the paravertebral area 5 cm on either side of the midline, but should be placed lateral to this area on the left and/or right sides. After a variable period of time, the tape and chambers are removed and the skin at the site of one set is irradiated with a UV source. At variable times after irradiation, usually multiples of 24 h, both test sites are then visually inspected and the strength of any reaction is recorded using a grading scale.

Treatment

For a photosensitive reaction to occur, both a photosensitizing substance and the requisite radiation must be present. The condition can be cured if one or other of these two triggers is removed from the equation. It is obviously much easier to eliminate the photosensitizer in question than to control the sun exposure.

General Measures

I. *Elimination of antigen*: Eliminating the topical agent or medicine responsible for the reaction should lead to a cure. With a systemic photosensitivity reaction, the suspected drug must be replaced with a medicine from another therapeutic class. For a photoallergic reaction, the medicinal product responsible must be identified and eliminated because not only will the rash spread to protected areas of skin, but it will also occur at low doses and after mild exposure. In patients presenting with a phototoxic reaction (dose-dependent, requiring intense UV exposure and a high concentration of the drug in the skin), the risk of phototoxicity can be attenuated by reducing the dose prescribed and changing the time of intake to the evening (to ensure that the concentration in the skin is lower during the day). It should be noted that photosensitivity does not decrease immediately the medication presumed responsible is withdrawn.

II. *Photoprotection:* Reducing exposure to radiation is the only solution when it has not been possible to identify the photoallergen or when the patient's life depends on the drug considered to be the source of the reaction. Such patients must avoid going out in the mid-day sun when UV irradiation is at its peak. Clothing providing sufficient protection against UV rays and a wide-brimmed hat must be worn. Protective clothing is much more effective than sun protection products, which must nonetheless also be used.

Filters are synthetic chemical substances which absorb either UVB rays or UVB and UVA rays. Since most photosensitivity reactions are triggered by UVAs, patients must be advised to use "Very High Protection 50+" products with the highest possible UVA protection factor. However, chemical filters may also cause contact photoallergic reactions. Patients presenting with medicinal product-related photosensitization should therefore be advised to use sun protection products containing physical screens only consisting of minute particles of titanium dioxide, zinc oxide or mica. Nonetheless, it is important to be aware of the limitations of sun protection products since, although they certainly reduce the level of irradiation absorbed by the skin, there are currently no products available on the market actually capable of preventing a photosensitivity reaction.

Specific Measures

Corticosteroids: Topical corticosteroids are used for treating localised forms. In severe ones, though, also depending on the extent of the affected skin, systemic corticosteroids may additionally be required.

Prevention

A list of days liable to induce phototoxic and photoallergic reactions (Table 5.1) can be used as a guide to eliminate at risk days. Photoallergic reactions are difficult to prevent since they depend on the immune status of the patient. Nonetheless, potentially phototoxic substances must be used with extreme caution during sunny periods. Patients must be told to avoid using fragrances and deodorants before going out into the sun.

CHRONIC ACTINIC DERMATITIS

Formerly known as persistent light reaction or actinic reticuloid syndrome, chronic actinic dermatitis is a rare photodermatitis generally affecting men aged over 50 who have worked outdoors.

Clinical Features

Clinically, it presents as a pruriginous, eczematiform rash developing on photo-exposed areas where, owing to its chronic nature, it gives the skin an infiltrated lichenified appearance, gradually spreading into the covered zones. This is a highly debilitating condition causing a severe reaction even to minimal exposure. The patient is allergic to UVBs, UVAs and even visible wavelengths. The patient can also be allergic to plants of the Asteraceae family, sesquiterpenic lactones, colophane, fragrances and certain sun filters.

Treatment

The results obtained with *topical treatments* are disappointing. The protection afforded by suncreams is insufficient, even when very high protection factor products are used, in preference those containing mineral screens only since many patients can also be allergic to chemical filters. Protective clothing is effective but is not appropriate for certain parts of the body such as the face and hands.

a. *PUVA therapy* is the first line treatment for severe forms but is often initially poorly tolerated. Before treatment is started, the UVA MED must be established using the light tubes that will later be used for the treatment sessions. The initial UVA dose delivered must be less than the UVA MED (i.e. very low, about 0.25 to 0.50 J/cm^2), and should then be gradually increased (by about 0.25 J/cm^2 at each session) depending on tolerance. Generally, a patient will have three sessions per week for a total of 10 weeks. Treatment can be stopped when light tolerance has reached an acceptable level, but if photosensitivity persists, maintenance treatment should be offered (one PUVA therapy session a week during the summer and one session every two weeks in winter).

A combination with steroids known as *Cortico-PUVA therapy* renders the first phototherapy sessions more bearable. The patient is given systemic corticosteroids at a dose of 1 mg/kg/day starting 8 days before PUVA therapy and continued at the same dose for 4 weeks and then gradually withdrawn.

b. Narrow band UVB phototherapy (TL01 tubes) has been used in some cases, starting at a dose well below the MED (about 10 to 20 mJ/cm^2) and gradually increasing the dose delivered.

c. *Immunosuppressants* are the second line treatment. These include cyclosporine 35–5 mg/kg, mycophenolate mofetil 25–40 mg/kg and azathioprine 1–2.5 mg/kg .

Bibliography

1. Eczema, in. Sardana k, Mahajan S, Garg VK. Diagnosis and Management of Skin Disorders: An Evidence-Based Approach, 1/e.: Lippincott Williams and Wilkins, 2012 (reprint 2015).

2. Fast Facts: Eczema and Contact Dermatitis By John Berth-Jones, Eunice Tan and Howard I Malbach Published 2004.

3. Thieme Clinical Companions Dermatology. Sterry, Dermatology© 2006 Thieme.

6

Airborne Contact Dermatitis

INTRODUCTION

Airborne contact dermatitis (ABCD) denotes an unique subtype of contact dermatitis that originates from dust, spray, pollens or volatile chemicals by airborne particles that settle on the exposed skin as well as body folds (Handa et al). This form of dermatitis commonly involves face, neck, V-area of chest, eyelids as well as nonexposed skin such as axilla and waist lines. Sometimes this form of dermatitis can be generalized (Gordon, Bajaj).

ABCD often cause diagnostic problems in terms of identifying the causative agent and the treatment is equally challenging. ABCD is clinically identified on the basis of history, morphology and distribution of lesions and proved by allergic patch test.

Incidence of airborne dermatoses has increased considerably during recent years (Huygens and Goossens). As per the previous reports by Nandakishor et al and Pasricha et al, ABCD in Indian patients has been attributed exclusively by pollens of plants like *Parthenium hysterophorus, Xanthium strumarium, Chrysanthemum coronarium, Helianthus annus and Dahlia pimrata.* The recent reports by Ghosh and Johnson et al have shown that the scenario has been changing rapidly in urban and semiurban perspective in developing countries where cement, perfumes, deodorants, volatile paints, etc. have become the commonest allergens contributing to ABCD.

In this chapter the various epidemiological aspects of ABCD, newly identified occupational and nonoccupational airborne contactants, clinical manifestations and treatment modalities available in ABCD will be discussed.

EPIDEMIOLOGY

Epidemiologically, ABCD can be classified into occupational and nonoccupational ABCD. It is believed that airborne irritant dermatitis is much common than the allergic type. Cabanillas et al reported a 3% prevalence of allergic ABCD to plant antigens among patients attending contact dermatitis unit. Sharma VK et al reported that in India Parthenium dermatitis caused by *Parthenium hysterophorus*, is an important cause of ABCD. In a study by Agarwal et al from South India, 50 patients of Parthenium dermatitis were studied. Among them 90% were farmer by occupation and lesions were aggravated in summer. The most common type of dermatitis was the classic ABCD pattern (46%), followed by mixed pattern (30%), erythroderma (14%) and chronic actinic dermatitis (10%).

In another study by Singhal et al 75 patients with clinically suspected contact dermatitis were patch tested with the Indian Standard Series and indigenous antigens. Parthenium was the most common contact sensitizer (20%) followed by potassium dichromate (16%), xanthium (13.3%), nickel sulphate (12%), chrysanthemum (8%) and mercaptobenzothiazole (6.7%).

PATHOGENESIS

In ABCD, on initial exposure to the antigen there is no response which is referred to as refractory phase. This is followed by an induction phase where the hapten penetrates the skin, conjugates with an epidermal protein and comes in contact with antigen presenting cells, migrates to the draining lymph nodes followed by stimulation of naïve T cells. This leads to proliferation of activated T cells to produce effector and memory cells which then enter the circulation. Reexposure to the specific hapten leads to the release of mediators producing skin inflammation (Lakshmi and Srinivas).

Causes

Antigens which cause ABCD (modified from Santos et al and Huygens et al) has been listed in Table 6.1.

CLINICAL FEATURES

A person may be sensitized to airborne contactants by direct and indirect contact or ingestion of allergens.

Table 6.1: Antigens contributing airborne contact dermatitis (ABCD)

Plants and natural resins	Plastics, rubber and glues	Metals	Industrial chemicals and drugs	Miscellaneous
Parthenium hysterophorus	Epoxy resins	Chromate	Organophosphorus pesticides	Agricultural dusts
Eucalyptus pulverulenta	Formaldehyde and formaldehyde resins	Cobalt	Animal feed antibiotics Paraphenylenediamine	Disperse dyes
Chrysanthemum Sunflower Garlic	Rubber additives Fragrance mix		Potassium metabisulphite Quaternerium-15 Potassium dichromate	
Essential oils Tropical and domestic woods Latex Psyllium	Colophony		Metaproterenol	

Dooms-Goossens and Deleu classified airborne dermatitis into 5 types:

1. Airborne irritant contact dermatitis
2. Airborne allergic contact dermatitis
3. Airborne phototoxic reactions
4. Airborne photoallergic reactions
5. Airborne contact urticaria

Some agents such as *P. hysterophorus* can produce both allergic CD and phototoxic reactions. Mixed pattern is also seen in formaldehyde and phosphorus sesquisulfide where allergic CD can coexist with contact urticaria (Dooms-Goossens and Deleu).

In classical ABCD there is involvement of the exposed areas of face (Figs 6.1 and 6.2), V-area of neck, hand and forearms, 'Wilkinson's triangle', eyelids, nasolabial folds and under the chin. Other than these, areas of skin where the dust and fibers can be trapped such as neck (under shirt collar) (Fig. 6.3), forearms (under cuffs) (Fig. 6.4), lower legs (inside trouser leg) can also be affected. Contact dermatitis from prolonged and repeated exposure to small quantities of airborne allergens such as pollens and dust may

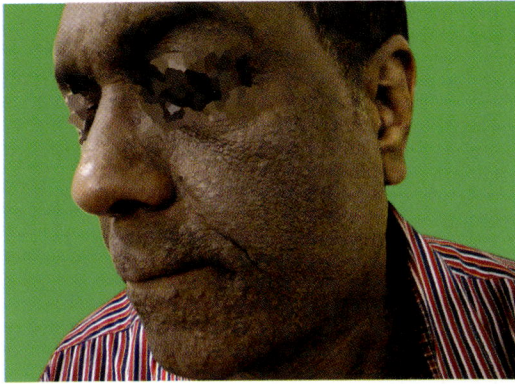

Fig. 6.1: Face affected by airborne contact dermatitis

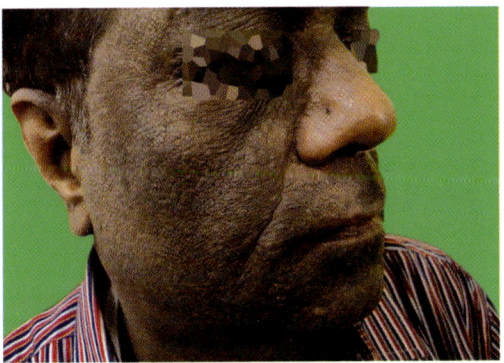

Fig. 6.2: Face (contralateral side) affected by airborne contact dermatitis

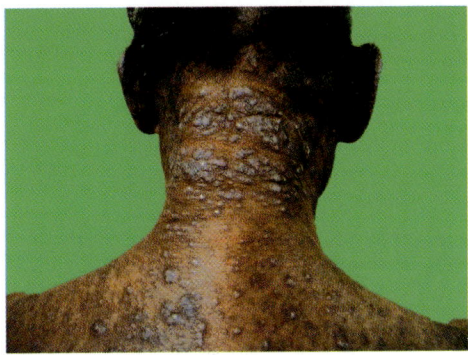

Fig. 6.3: Nape of the neck and upper back affected by airborne contact dermatitis

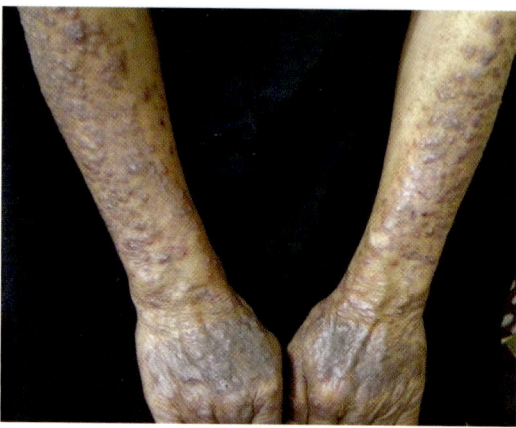

Fig. 6.4: Forearm affected by airborne contact dermatitis

produce diffuse, dry and lichenified eruptions. The most commonly seen parthenium dermatitis classically presents as ABCD but may occasionally present with photosensitive lichenoid eruptions. ABCD and photoallergic dermatitis have similar presentation as both photoexposed and covered areas are involved in ABCD (Sharma and Sethuraman). However, in photoallergic dermatitis usually submental and post-auricular area is usually spared (Ghosh) (Figs 6.5 and 6.6). Sawdust from teak and mahogany contain sensitizers that produce a dry dermatitis of face, penis and scrotum of carpenters (Sharma and Sethuraman).

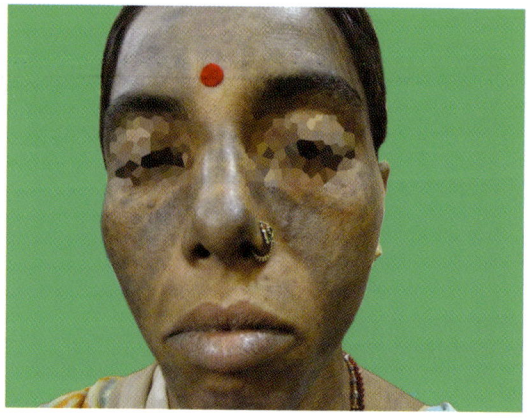

Fig. 6.5: A female patient affected by airborne contact dermatitis

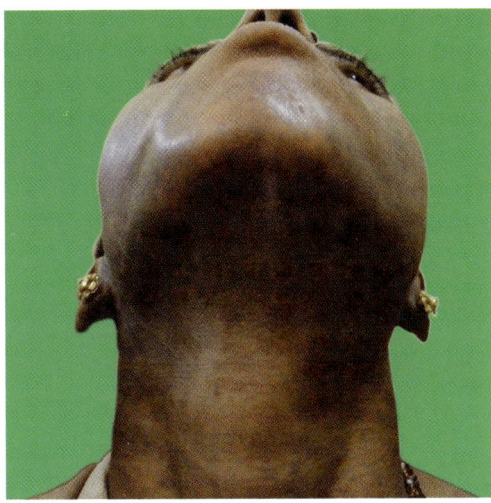

Fig. 6.6: Submental area affected by airborne contact dermatitis (*cf.* Photoallergic dermatitis)

Cement dust usually presents as a dry, lichenified dermatitis due to the presence of chromates. Household sprays, insecticides and occupational volatile chemicals can produce eyelid dermatitis (Rietschel and Fowler). Airborne chloromethyl and methylisothiazolinone dermatitis may appear in face of sensitized individuals who stay in newly painted rooms (Bohn, Niederer, Brehm et al). Airborne contact urticaria can be associated with rhinitis, conjunctivitis and asthma in patients with hypersensitivity to latex proteins in rubber gloves (Christophe, Le, Ducombs). Airborne transmission of latex allergens is enhanced by their adsorption onto the cornstarch. Airborne contact urticaria is also reported in person exposed to cinchona dust (Dooms-Goossens).

DIAGNOSIS

After clinically suspecting a case as ABCD, it needs to be confirmed with patch test or prick test. The patch test is used to find the causative allergens. In case of volatile allergens high dilution should be used during patch test as there is a chance of developing irritant reaction. For testing wood dust, it should not be moistened as it increases irritancy. Photopatch test can be used for excluding light as a precipitating factor.

In a study by Green and Ferguson sesquiterpene lactone (SL) mix detected only 35% of Compositae allergy and hence not a very useful screening test. These patients could be diagnosed by additional Compositae mix and hence more useful.

TREATMENT

Treatment of ABCD can be broadly divided into:

- Preventive management
- Treatment of existing dermatitis

Preventive Management

In cases of ABCD due to Parthenium, one should avoid going outdoors on days when pollen are present in high concentration specially in summers and in the month of September to November. Airconditioning also decreases indoor pollen load. Simple routine like taking a bath after coming indoors, wearing fresh clothes and eliminating grasses and weeds in the house garden can be of great benefit. Other preventive measures include photoprotection, change of job and residence, if possible (Nicholson, Llewellyn, English). In some countries, addition of ferrous sulphate to cement converts the hexavalent chromates into trivalent ones and thereby reducing the sensitizing potential.

Treatment of Existing Dermatitis

Topical

- Topical steroids are the mainstay of therapy.
- Emollients can be co-prescribed in lichenified lesions whereas in oozing lesions drying agents such as aluminum sulfate and calcium acetate can be given.

Systemic

- Systemic steroids are indicated when more than 25% of body surface area is involved.
- Psoralens and UVA
- UVB
- In a therapeutic study of patients with Parthenium dermatitis treated with azathioprine was given as weekly pulse dose (Verma KK et al)

- Parthenium dermatitis, unresponsive to topical treatment has been treated with oral methotrexate in a dose of 15 mg/week (Sharma et al)
- Handa et al evaluated the effect of oral hyposensitization as an alternative therapeutic modality and observed a gradual improvement in the clinical status of 70% of those patients who completed the study.

CONCLUSION

Evidence indicates that up to 50% of patients with ABCD experience adverse effects on quality of life, daily function and personal relationship and take time off work on sick leave because of their skin disease. It is emphasized that avoidance of further exposure can lead to recovery from dermatitis in many cases. With respect to ABCD secondary to Parthenium dermatitis, there are continuing attempts to control the spread of weed through biological measures like introduction of exotic arthropods, use of antagonistic plants and bioherbicides as well as selective chemical herbicides

Bibliography

1. Agarwal KK, Souza MD. Airborne contact dermatitis induced by parthenium:A study of 50 cases in South India. Clin Exp Dermatol 2009;34:e4–6.

2. Bajaj AK.Contact dermatitis.In IADVL Textbook and Atlas of Dermatology. In:Valia RG, Editor, 2nd Ed, Vol 1. Mumbai: Bhalani; 2001, p.453–97.

3. Bohn S, Niederer M, Brehm K, et al. Airborne contact dermatitis from methylchloroisothiazolinone in wall paint. Abolition of symptoms by chemical allergen inactivation. Contact Dermatitis 2003;31:275–6.

4. Cabanillas M, Fernandez-Redondo V, Toribio J. Allergic contact dermatitis to plants in a Spanish dermatology department: A 7-year review. Contact Dermatitis 2006;55:84–91.

5. Christophe J, Le Coz, Ducombs G. Plants and plant product contact dermatitis. In: Frosch PJ, Menne T, Lepoittevin JP, Editors, 4th ed. Heidelberg: Springer; 2006. p.751–800.

6. Dooms-Goossens A, Deleu H. Airborne contact dermatitis: An update. Contact Dermatitis 1991;25:211–7.

7. Dooms-Goossens A, Deveylder H, Duron C, et al. Airborne contact urticaria due to cinchona. Contact Dermatitis 1986;15:258.

8. Ghosh S. Airborne contact dermatitis of non-plant origin: An overview. Ind J Dermatol 2011;56:(6)711–4.

9. Ghosh S. Airborne contact dermatitis: An urban perspective. Perils of urban pollution: Proceedings National Seminar on Pollution in Urban Industrial Environment. In:Mitra AK, Editor. Kolkata: St Xavier's College; 2006 P. 9–12.

10. Ghosh S. Atlas and Synopsis of Contact and Occupational Dermatology. Jaypee Brothers New Delhi 2008:20–4.

11. Gordon LA. Compositae dermatitis. Australas J Dermatol 1999;40: 123–30.

12. Green C, Ferguson J. Sesquiterpene lactone mix is not an adequate screen for Compositae allergy. Contact Dermatitis 1994;31:151–3.

13. Handa F, Handa S, Handa R. Environmental factors and the skin. In:Valia RG, Editor.IADVL Textbook and Atlas of Dermatology. 2nd ed, Vol.1. Mumbai: Bhalani; 2001; p 81–91.

14. Handa S, Sahoo B, Sharma VK. Oral hyposensitisation in patients with contact dermatitis from *Parthenium hysterophorus*. Contact Dermatitis 2001; 44:279–82.

15. Huygen S, Goossen A. An update on airborne contact dermatitis. Contact Dermatitis 2001;44:1–6.

16. Lakshmi C, Srinivas CR. Parthenium dermatitis caused by immediate and delayed hypersensitivity. Contact Dermatitis 2007;57:64–5.

17. Nandakishore TH, Pasricha JS. Pattern of cross-sensitivity between four Compositae plants *Parthenium hysterophorus, Xanthium strumarium, Chrysanthemum coronarium, Helianthus annus* in Indian patients. Contact Dermatitis 1994;30:162–7.

18. Nicholson PJ, Llewellyn D, English JS. On behalf of the Guidelines Development Group. Evidence-based guidelines for the prevention, identification and management of occupational contact dermatitis and urticaria. Contact Dermatitis 2010;63:177–86.

19. Pasricha JS, Verma KK, D'souza P. Airborne contact dermatitis caused exclusively by *Xanthium strumarium*. Indian J Dermatol Venerol Leprol 1995;61:354–5.

20. Rietschel RL, Fowler JF. Fisher's Contact Dermatitis. Hamilton: BC Decker Inc; 2008, p. 69–101.

21. Santos R, Goossens AR. An update on airborne contact dermatitis: 2001–2006. Contact Dermatitis 2007;57:353–60.

22. Sharma VK, Bhat R, Sethuraman G, et al. Treatment of parthenium dermatitis with methotrexate. Contact Dermatitis 2007; 57:118–9.

23. Sharma VK, Sethuraman G, Bhat R. Evaluation of clinical patterns of Parthenium dermatitis: A study of 74 cases. Contact Dermatitis 2005;44: 49–50.

24. Sharma VK, Sethuraman G, Tejasvi T. Comparison of patch test contact sensitivity to acetone and aqueous extracts of *Parthenium hysterophorus* in patients with airborne contact dermatitis. Contact Dermatitis 2004;50:230–2.

25. Sharma VK, Sethuraman G. Parthenium dermatitis. Dermatitis 2007;18:183–90.

26. Singhal V, Reddy BS. Common contact sensitizers in Delhi. J Dermatol 2000;27:440–5.

27. Verma KK, Bansal A, Sethuraman G. Parthenium dermatitis treated with azathioprine weekly pulse doses. Indian J Dermatol Venereol Leprol 2006;72:24–7.

7

Diaper Dermatitis

INTRODUCTION

Diaper dermatitis also known as napkin dermatitis, nappy rash or diaper rash is one of the most common skin conditions affecting neonates and infants. Classically, the term is used to describe irritant contact dermatitis of the diaper area and needs to be differentiated from other dermatoses that can affect that area.

PATHOGENESIS

Prolonged contact with a mixture of urine and faces is central to the pathogenesis of diaper dermatitis (Scheinfeld et al). Presence of urine produces excessive hydration and subsequent maceration of the skin of the anogenital region predisposing this area to effects of friction by the diaper. Overhydration also impairs the barrier function of the skin increasing its permeability for various irritants. Fecal contamination leads to breakdown of urea present in urine to ammonia that increases the pH of skin. This promotes the activity of various fecal enzymes such as proteases, ureases and lipases, that subsequently increases the permeability of skin and render it susceptible to irritant action of bile salts and acids. Exposure to such irritants under occlusion for a prolonged period of time leads to epidermal barrier disruption and erythema of skin (Scheinfeld et al).

The incidence of diaper dermatitis is related inversely to frequency of diaper change and directly to frequency of bowel movements and presence of diarrhea (Jordan et al, Adalat et al). Exclusively breastfeeding infants have a lower incidence of moderate to severe diaper dermatitis as compared to formula fed infants possibly due to lower stool pH and enzyme activity in former (Berg et al, Jordan et al, Pratt et al). No difference has been found in the flora of skin of diaper area of infants wearing disposable diapers with cellulose pulp core with or without absorbent gel material and cloth diapers (Keswick et al). However, candidal superinfection is a common cause of persistence of inflammation in the diaper area and should be excluded in every diaper dermatitis that lasts beyond 48–72 hours (Murat-Susiæ et al, Shin et al). Irritant diaper dermatitis usually resolves when the child becomes toilet trained.

CLINICAL FEATURES

The most common presentation is irritant contact diaper dermatitis (IDD) typically affecting convex areas of buttocks and perianal areas, mons pubis, upper thighs, lower abdomen, scrotum and outer surface of labia majora (Fig. 7.1). The sites with maximum contact with the diaper have the greatest severity of lesions. Inguinal folds are spared in classical IDD due to disposable diapers as they are protected from contents of the diaper. It initially presents as localized sharply demarcated mildly scaly erythema that may progress to painful confluent erythema, erosions and frank ulceration. Regression of lesions leaves wrinkled skin resembling cigarette paper.

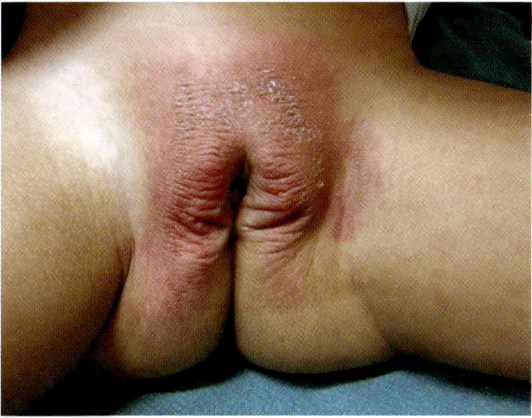

Fig. 7.1: Irritant diaper dermatitis affecting the convex surfaces of labia majora and mons pubis while sparing the vulva and inguinal folds

In a Chinese study, where cloth diapers are being used found IDD to be rare in buttocks or genitalia but common in perianal and intertriginous areas possibly due to accumulation or residual collection of mixture of urine and feces trickling into the inguinal folds as cloth diapers have minimum absorptive and holding capacity (Liu et al). The typically erosive form with crater-like punched out erosions and ulcerations with heaped up borders affecting the perianal areas, glans penis or urinary meatus is known as Jacquet dermatitis occurs due to infrequent diaper changes compounded by frequent liquid stools (Bluestein et al). Pseudo-verrucous papules and nodules present with shiny, smooth, flat topped moist or ulcerated papules (Fig. 7.2) while granuloma gluteale infantum presents with large violaceous papules and nodules with erosions over the buttocks, lower abdomen, groin, penis and even axillae and neck. The name granuloma gluteale infantum is a misnomer as no granulomas are found histo-pathologically and the condition is basically an IDD aggravated due to repeated and prolonged application of topical steroids and Candida superinfection (Murat-Susiæ et al, Scheinfeld et al, Humphrey et al). It is usually self limiting, resolving in a few weeks to months often with residual scarring (Shin et al, Bluestein et al). Diaper dermatitis may also lead to id eruption occurring beyond the diaper area (Rattet et al) (Fig. 7.3).

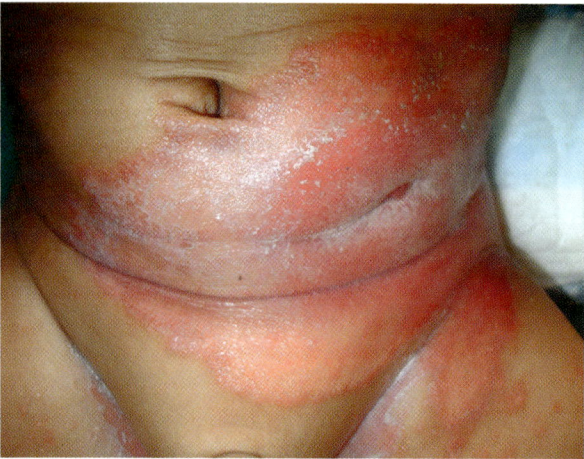

Fig. 7.2: Jacquet dermatitis

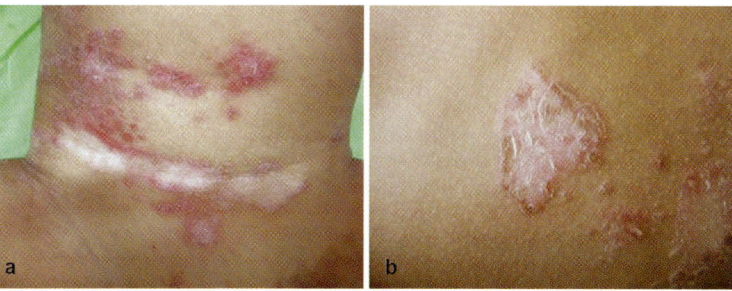

Fig. 7.3: (a) Psoriasiform id secondary to diaper dermatitis; (b) Close up view

DIFFERENTIAL DIAGNOSIS

IDD needs to be differentiated from other conditions that affect the diaper area (Table 7.1). *Candida albicans* is a frequent secondary offender and leads to worsening of the pre-existing diaper dermatitis (Fig. 7.4). Severe chronic candidal diaper dermatitis and napkin dermatitis may sometimes indicate underlying immunodeficiency including HIV (Thiboutot et al). Allergic contact dermatitis is rare in children less than 2 years due to the incompletely developed immune response.

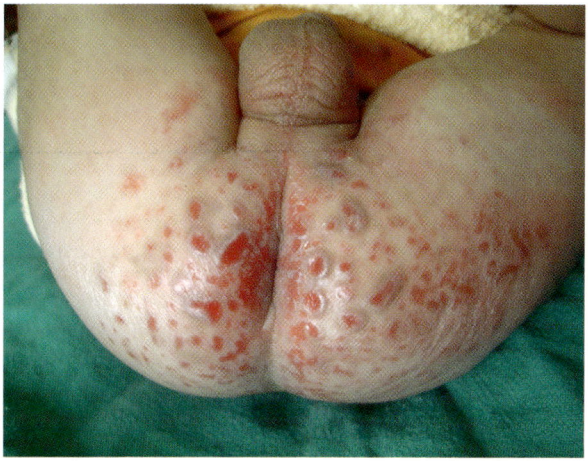

Fig. 7.4: Irritant diaper dermatitis around a urostomy in an infant secondarily complicated by candidiasis

Table 7.1: Differential diagnosis of diaper dermatitis (Coughlin et al, Scheinfeld et al, Shin et al, Humphrey et al, Morris et al)

	Clinical features	Site
Candidiasis	Beefy red plaques with satellite papules and pustules	Diapered skin with accentuation in perianal area, inguinal folds and scrotum
Dermatophytosis	Erythematous scaly annular plaques with central clearing (Fig. 7.5)	Any part of anogenital region
Streptococcal perianal dermatitis	Sharply demarcated fiery red patches, some maceration, pain, low grade fever, malaise, painful defecation	Perianal, inguinal areas
Allergic contact dermatitis	Eczematous, pruritic eruption with redness, edema, vesicles and superficial erosions	Waistline and upper thighs (area in contact with elastic components of diaper) and diaper closure area (glue)
Infantile seborrheic	Well demarcated erythematous patches with or without yellow or greasy scale, cradle cap (Fig. 7.6)	Inguinal, axillary folds, neck
Atopic dermatitis	Usually spares the anogenital area, if present lesions are pruritic and involvement is recurrent and resistant	Typical lesions present on other areas according to age of the child
Napkin psoriasis	Sharply demarcated, erythematous plaques without typical scales, usually first site of involvement in children due to koebnerisation	Skin folds, gluteal cleft
Acrodermatitis enteropathica	Sharply demarcated eruption with crusting, erosions, pustules with accentuated scale at margin, alopecia and diarrhea	Acral, peri-orificial and anogenital distribution
Langerhans cell histiocytosis	Eczematous eruption with greasy scaling, crusting with reddish brown or yellow hemorrhagic papules resembling petechiae with atrophy and deep ulceration	Inguinal folds, postauricular areas

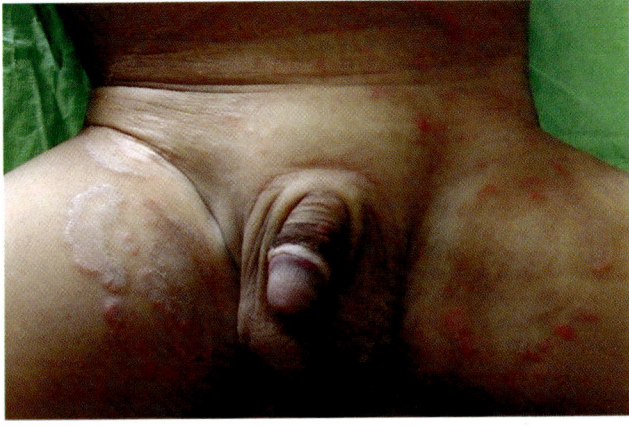

Fig. 7.5: Dermatophytosis affecting the diaper area

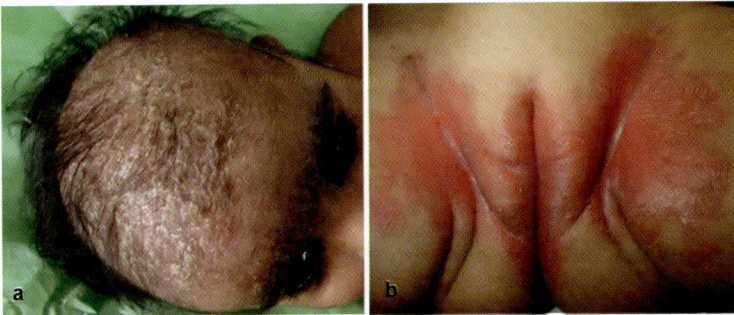

Fig. 7.6: (a) Cradle cap in infant with seborrheic dermatitis; (b)Seborrheic dermatitis with greasy scales affecting the inguinal region

MANAGEMENT

The basic regime to be followed in treatment of IDD can be remembered by the Mnemonic ABCDE: A for air or time without diaper, B for barrier cream, C for cleansing/corticosteroids, D for diaper to be used, E for education of the parents (Boiko et al). Aeration of the skin possibly when the infant is sleeping or just after urination and defecation provides respite from the frictional and irritant effects of the wet diaper fabric. Barrier preparations such as generic preservative free zinc oxide ointment or paste are effective for preventing and even treating mild IDD. Barrier creams may include petrolatum, cord liver oil, dimethicone, lanolin, white soft paraffin and titanium oxide (Ward et al). These need to be applied generously at each diaper change and may be covered with petrolatum to avoid sticking to the diaper (Borowski et al). They create a lipid film over the surface of skin to protect the skin from friction, irritants and micro-organisms and their lipids penetrate into the stratum corneum, assuming the role of endogenous lipids and preventing excessive water loss (Atherton et al, Shin et al). Ointments and pastes are more effective than oils, creams and lotions as the latter do not adhere that well to denuded skin and may contain preservatives. Topical vitamin A has been shown to be ineffective for prevention or treatment of IDD (Davies et al, Bosch-Banyeras et al). Products containing fragrances and additives such as vitamins, boric acid, camphor, phenol, salicylates and baking soda should be avoided. Corn starch is effective in protecting from frictional injury and preventing growth of *Candida albicans* (Leyden et al). Powders should be used with care to prevent aspiration pneumonitis and talc should be avoided.

Cleansing

Avoidance of harsh scrubbing or overcleansing should be stressed taking due care to ensure that no urine or fecal residue is left in creases and folds. When using a disposable diaper, minimal cleansing is required after urination. Gentle cleansing with warm water and a mild cleanser should be carried out if the diaper area is soiled. Any residual adherent barrier paste does not need to be wiped off at each diaper change except after defecation for which mineral oil on a cotton-ball may be used. Cleansing agents with a high pH can adversely affect the skin barrier and use of syndets that have near physiologic pH is recommended (Lund et al, Blume-Peytavi et al, Klunk et al). Present day wipes are alcohol-free soft cloth like wipes with low abrasion potential and non-ionic surfactants (Odio et al, Manzini et al). Use of disposable wipes do not have any adverse effect on transepidermal water loss, skin pH, erythema or microbial flora as compared to cotton wool and water (Lavender et al) and is safe even in infants with atopic dermatitis (Ehretsmann et al). Wipes should not be used on eroded or ulcerated skin. Allergic contact dermatitis has been reported to the preservative methylisothiazolinone present in disposable wipes (Chang et al).

The risk of IDD is dependent on type of diaper worn, length of time the diaper is worn and the frequency of diaper change. Ideally, diaper should be changed after every urination and defecation. This would mean changing the diaper every 1–2 hours in neonates with high wetting frequency and every 3–4 hours in other infants during daytime and at least once during the night. A diaper slightly larger than the infants size is preferable to minimize effect of frictional and irritant factors. Early diapers had a cellulose fluff and impenetrable outer cover to prevent leakage of fluids that led to increased humidity and skin maceration. Present day disposable diapers have an absorbent gelling material (AGM) core containing cross-linked sodium polyacrylate polymers that can absorb more than 80 times its weight in liquid and outermost layer made of polypropylene that is permeable to air and vapor but impermeable to fluids. The AGM core binds water in a gel matrix away from the skin reducing skin wetting, mixing of urine and feces and achieving better pH control and are less likely to cause IDD as compared to conventional disposable or cloth diapers (Akin et al, Campbell et al, Davis et al). However, such superabsorbent diapers can also lead to IDD, if left in place for too long. Cloth diapers are not advisable for infants with IDD as they increase skin wetness and allow mixing of urine and feces.

In cases with severe symptoms or persisting symptoms despite conservative therapy, hydrocortisone 1% cream can be applied sparingly to the affected area before barrier cream for not more than 2 weeks unless under supervision of a dermatologist. Mid-to-high potency steroids should never be used in the diaper area as they can lead to atrophy, candidiasis, granuloma gluteale infantum and significant systemic absorption due to presence of moisture, occlusive diapers and higher body surface area to volume ratio in infants. Tacrolimus and other calcineurin inhibitors can be used as steroid sparing agents (Patel et al). Antifungal creams such as clotrimazole, ketoconazole and miconazole may be used when there is superinfection with Candida or in any IDD that lasts longer than a few days and requires at least mild topical steroids to control infection. Application should be continued till at least 1 week after clearance of the eruption.

Bibliography

1. Adalat S, Wall D, Goodyear H. Diaper dermatitis—frequency and contributory factors in hospital attending children. Pediatr Dermatol 2007;24:483–8.

2. Akin F, Spraker M, Aly R, Leyden J, Raynor W, Landin W. Effects of breathable disposable diapers: reduced prevalence of Candida and common diaper dermatitis. Pediatr Dermatol 2001;18:282–90.

3. Atherton DJ. A review of the pathophysiology, prevention and treatment of irritant diaper dermatitis. Curr Med Res Opin 2004;20:645–9.

4. Berg RW, Buckingham KW, Stewart RL. Etiologic factors in diaper dermatitis: the role of urine. Pediatr Dermatol 1986;3:102–6.

5. Bluestein J, Furner BB, Phillips D. Granuloma gluteale infantum: case report and review of the literature. Pediatr Dermatol 1990;7:196–8.

6. Blume-Peytavi U, Cork MJ, Faergemann J Szczapa J, Vanaclocha F, Gelmetti C. Bathing and cleansing in newborns from day 1 to first year of life: recommendations from a European round table meeting. J Eur Acad Dermatol Venereol 2009;23:751–759.

7. Boiko S. Treatment of diaper dermatitis. Dermatol Clin. 1999;17:235–40.

8. Borkowski S. Diaper rash care and management. Pediatr Nurse 2004; 30:467–70.

9. Bosch-Banyeras JM, Catala M, Mas P, Simon JL, Puig A. Diaper dermatitis. Value of vitamin A topically applied. Clin Pediatr 1988;27:448–50.

10. Campbell RL, Bartlett AV, Sarbaugh FC, Pickering LK. Effects of diaper types on diaper dermatitis associated with diarrhea and antibiotic use in children in day-care centers. Pediatr Dermatol 1988;5:83–87.

11. Chang MW, Nakrani R. Six children with allergic contact dermatitis to methylisothiazolinone in wet wipes (baby wipes). Pediatrics 2014;133: e434–e438.

12. Coughlin CC, Eichenfield LF, Frieden IJ. Diaper dermatitis: clinical characteristics and differential diagnosis. Pediatr Dermatol. 2014;31 Suppl 1:19–24.

13. Davies MW, Dore AJ, Perissinotto KL. Topical vitamin A, or its derivatives, for treating and preventing napkin dermatitis in infants. Cochrane Database Syst Rev 2005:19;4:CD004300.

14. Davis JA, Leyden JJ, Grove GL, Raynor WJ. Comparison of disposable diapers with fluff absorbent and fluff plus absorbent polymers: effects on skin hydration, skin pH, and diaper dermatitis. Pediatr Dermatol 1989;6:102–108.

15. Ehretsmann C, Schaefer P, Adam R. Cutaneous tolerance of baby wipes by infants with atopic dermatitis, and comparison of the mildness of baby wipe and water in infant skin. J Eur Acad Dermatol Venereol 2001;15(Suppl 1):16–21.

16. Humphrey S, Bergman JN, Au S. Practical Management Strategies for Diaper Dermatitis. Skin Therapy Letter 2006;11:1–6.

17. Jordan WE, Lawson KD, Berg RW, Franxman JJ, Marrer AM. Diaper dermatitis: frequency and severity among a general infant population. Pediatr Dermatol 1986;3:198–207.

18. Keswick BH, Seymour JL, Milligan MC. Diaper area skin microflora of normal children and children with atopic dermatitis. J Clin Microbiol 1987;25:216–221.

19. Klunk C, Domingues E, Wiss K. Update on Diaper Dermatitis. Clin Dermatology. 2014;32:477–87.

20. Lavender T, Furber C, Campbell M, et al. Effect on skin hydration of using baby wipes to clean the napkin area of newborn babies: assessor-blinded randomised controlled equivalence trial. BMC Pediatr 2012;12:59.

21. Leyden JJ. Cornstarch, *Candida albicans*, and diaper rash. Pediatr Dermatol.1984;1:322–5.

22. Liu N, Wang X, Odio M. Frequency and severity of diaper dermatitis with use of traditional Chinese cloth diapers: observations in 3- to 9-month-old children. Pediatr Dermatol 2011;28:380–6.

23. Lund C. Prevention and management of infant skin breakdown. Nurs Clin North Am 1999;34:907–920.

24. Manzini BM, Ferdani G, Simonetti V, Donini M, Seidenari S.Contact sensitization in children. Pediatr Dermatol 1998;15:12–17.

25. Morris A, Rogers M, Fischer G, Williams K. Childhood psoriasis: a clinical review of 1262 cases. Pediatr Dermatol 2001;18:188–98.

26. Murat-Susiæ S, Husar K. Differential diagnosis of skin lesions in the diaper area. Acta Dermatovenerol Croat. 2007;15:108–12.

27. Odio M, Friedlander SF. Diaper dermatitis and advances in diaper technology. Curr Opin Pediatr 2000;12:342–346.

28. Patel RR, Vander Straten MR, Korman NJ. The safety and efficacy of tacrolimus therapy in patients younger than 2 years with atopic dermatitis. Arch Dermatol 2003;139:118–46.

29. Pratt AG, Reed WT Jr. Influence of the type of feeding on pH of stool, pH of skin and the incidence of perianal dermatitis in the newborn infant. J Pediatr 1955;46:539–43.

30. Rattet JP, Headley JL, Barr RJ. Diaper dermatitis with psoriasiform ID eruption. Int J Dermatol 1981;20:122–5.

31. Scheinfeld N. Diaper dermatitis: a review and brief survey of eruptions of the diaper area. Am J Clin Dermatol 2005;6:273–81.

32. Shin HT. Diagnosis and management of diaper dermatitis. Pediatr Clin North Am 2014;61:367–82.

33. Shin HT. Diaper dermatitis that does not quit. Dermatol Ther 2005;18:124–35.

34. Thiboutot DM, Beckford A, Mart CR, Sexton M, Maloney ME. Cytomegalovirus diaper dermatitis. Arch Dermatol 1991;127:396–8.

35. Ward DB, Fleischer AB, Feldman SR, Krowchuk DP. Characterization of diaper dermatitis in the United States. Arch Pediatr Adolesc Med 2000; 154: 943–946.

8

Atopic Dermatitis

DEFINITION AND INTRODUCTION

Atopic dermatitis (AD) is an acquired, chronic, inflammatory, pruritic skin disease of unknown origin that usually starts in early infancy (an adult-onset variant is recognized) with remissions and exacerbations; it is characterized by pruritus, eczematous lesions, xerosis (dry skin), and lichenification (thickening of the skin and an increase in skin markings).

It is frequently associated with abnormalities in skin barrier function, allergen sensitization, and recurrent skin infections.

AD is a complex genetic disease with underlying epithelial barrier defect involving skin as well as mucosa hence is often accompanied by other atopic disorders such as allergic rhinoconjunctivitis and asthma. These conditions may appear simultaneously or develop in succession. AD has a predilection for infants and young children, while asthma favors older children and pollen allergy predominates in adolescents. This characteristic age-dependent sequence is referred to as the **"atopic march"** (Asher et al, Williams et al).

EPIDEMIOLOGY

Since the 1960s, there has been a more than threefold increase in the prevalence of AD worldwide (Eichenfield LF et al). Prevalence rates in different geographical regions vary from as low as 1% to as high as 20% with higher prevalence in developed countries than developing countries. In general, the prevalence of AD in rural areas and low income countries is significantly lower than in their urban and high income counterparts, suggesting the importance of lifestyle and environment in expression of atopic disease. Factors traditionally associated with increased prevalence of AD include higher socioeconomic status, higher level of education, evolution of smaller families and increased urbanization (DaVeiga SP).

This observation supports the **hygiene hypothesis**, that allergic diseases might be prevented by "infection in early childhood transmitted by unhygienic contact with older siblings" (Strachan DP).

Prevalence of AD in Indian subcontinent is 3–4.2% and in general prevalence is increasing based on hospital data (Kanwar AJ).

PATHOGENESIS

Previously AD was thought to be a disease primarily mediated by immune system dysfunction, however, recently our understanding of AD has been changed with main focus on genetically mediated barrier abnormalities rather than immune dysregulation.

Large body of evidence now suggests that AD may be a disease of primary barrier failure, including defective stratum corneum permeability and antimicrobial defences which results in sustained and epicutaneous allergen penetration, leading to immune system activation and the resultant inflammation and pruritus that are typical of AD. The inappropriate activation of immune system results in further barrier disruption (Fig. 8.1) [Elias PM et al].

1. Genetics

Eighty percent of identical twins show concordance for AD. A child is at increased risk of developing AD if either parent is affected.

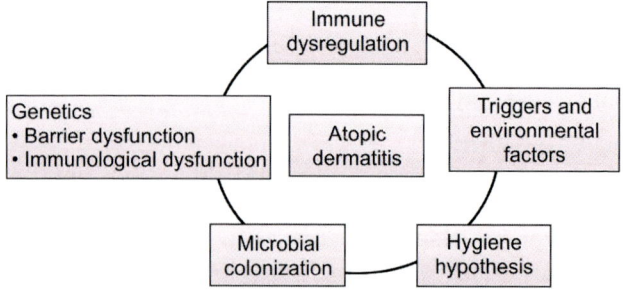

Fig. 8.1: Interplay of various factors that determine the manifestation of atopic dermatitis

2. Barrier Dysfunction

Mutations in the filaggrin gene (FLG), which encodes a protein that aggregates keratin filaments during terminal differentiation of the epidermis, are responsible for ichthyosis vulgaris and represent a major predisposing factor for AD. FLG mutations are associated with AD that presents early in life, tends to persist into childhood and adulthood, and is associated with wheezing in infancy and with asthma. FLG mutations are also associated with allergic rhinitis and keratosis pilaris, independent of AD. Hyperlinear palms are strongly associated with FLG mutations, with a 71% positive predictive value (PPV) for marked palmar hyperlinearity. However, not all the patients with AD have filaggrin gene defect. Marked decrease in skin barrier function also occurs due to the downregulation of cornified envelope genes (filaggrin and loricrin), reduced ceramide levels, increased levels of endogenous proteolytic enzymes, and enhanced transepidermal water loss (Bratton DL et al, Toda M et al).

This barrier dysfunction leads to increased allergen penetration into skin and increased microbial colonization and predisposes the affected individual to food allergies and respiratory allergies.

3. Defects in Adaptive and Immune Response Genes

Genetic defects responsible for immunological dysregulation are responsible for antigen presentation, cell mediated and humoral immune response and cell signalling in skin, e.g. CD-14, IL-4, IL-5, IL-13, toll like receptors, etc.

4. Immune Dysregulation

Not all cases of AD are associated with FLG mutations. AD patients often demonstrate immunologic features. T helper 2 (Th2) cytokines (e.g. IL-4, IL-5, IL-13) predominate in acute AD lesions while Th1 cytokines (IL-12 and IFN-γ predominate in chronic AD lesions.

Acute AD is associated with the production of T helper 2 (Th2) type cytokines, notably IL-4 and IL-13, which mediate immunoglobulin isotype switching to IgE synthesis and upregulate expression of adhesion molecules on endothelial cells.

In chronic AD, there is an increase in the production of IL-5, which is involved in eosinophil development and survival. Increased production of granulocyte macrophage colony-stimulating factor in AD inhibits apoptosis of monocytes, thereby contributing to the persistence of AD. The maintenance of chronic AD also involves production of the Th1-like cytokines IL-12 and IL-18, as well as several remodeling-associated cytokines, including IL-11 and transforming growth factor-1 (Toda M et al).

5. Microbial Colonization in AD

Various factors as epidermal barrier defects, reduction in antimicrobial peptides, toll-like receptors defects, decreased neutrophils recruitment to the skin and increased IgE levels contribute to increased microbial colonization and recurrent infections of skin.

Staphylococcus aureus colonization of the skin occurs in >90% of AD patients (Cho SH et al). *S. aureus* contributes to sensitization and inflammation in AD via several mechanisms such as TLR-2 recognition of *S. aureus* cell wall components (e.g. lipoteichoic acid, peptidoglycan) stimulates an inflammatory response, which staphylococcal superantigens amplify inflammatory reactions via multiple pathways (Cardona ID et al) and may contribute to corticosteroid resistance by inducing the competing β isoform of the glucocorticoid receptor, staphylococcal enterotoxins A-D (SEA-D) can provoke IgE-mediated sensitization, which also correlates with disease severity (Bunikowski R et al).

Malassezia is colonized in 100% AD patients and Malassezia spp are capable of activating mast cells, and inducing the Malassezia specific IgEs thereby contributing to the inflammation in AD. Patients with AD lesions on head, neck and upper trunk tend to respond to anti-Malassezia measures (Barker JN et al).

Triggers

Various environmental and other factors are known to worsen AD. Some of them are:

1. Changes in temperature
2. Sweating
3. Decrease in humidity
4. Contact with irritants as wool, chemicals, cosmetics, soaps, cigarette smoke.
5. Aeroallergens such as house dust mite, pollen, molds, pet dander, human dander.

6. Food allergens (eggs, peanuts, milk, fish, soy, wheat.

7. Emotional stress

8. Hormones (menstrual cycle and pregnancy)

CLINICAL FEATURES

Atopic dermatitis can be divided into three stages: Infantile AD, occurring from 2 months to 2 years of age; childhood AD, from 2 to 10 years; and adolescent/adult AD. In each stage, patients may develop acute, subacute and chronic eczematous lesions, all of which are intensely pruritic and often excoriated. AD typically begins during infancy. Approximately 50% of patients develop this illness by the first year of life and an additional 30% between the ages of 1–5 years. Between 50 and 80% of patients with AD develop allergic rhinitis or asthma later in childhood. Many of these patients outgrow their AD as they are developing respiratory allergy.

In all stages, pruritus is the hallmark. Itching often precedes the appearance of lesions; thus the concept that AD is "**the itch that rashes**." Pruritus may be intermittent throughout the day but is usually worse in the early evening and night. Its consequences are scratching, prurigo papules, lichenification, and eczematous skin lesions.

Acute lesions predominate in infantile AD and are characterized by edematous, erythematous papules and plaques that may exhibit vesiculation, oozing and serous crusting.

Subacute eczematous lesions display erythema, scaling and variable crusting.

Chronic lesions, which typify adolescent/adult AD, present as thickened plaques with lichenification as well as scale; prurigo nodularis like lesions can also develop. Perifollicular accentuation, and small, flat-topped papules (papular eczema) are particularly common in individuals with darkly pigmented skin. In any stage of AD, the most severely affected individuals may evolve to a generalized exfoliative erythroderma. All types of AD lesions can leave postinflammatory hyper-, hypo- or (in more severe cases) depigmentation upon resolution.

At all stages of AD, patients usually have dry, lackluster skin. A depiction of the sites of involvement in different age groups is given in (Fig. 8.2).

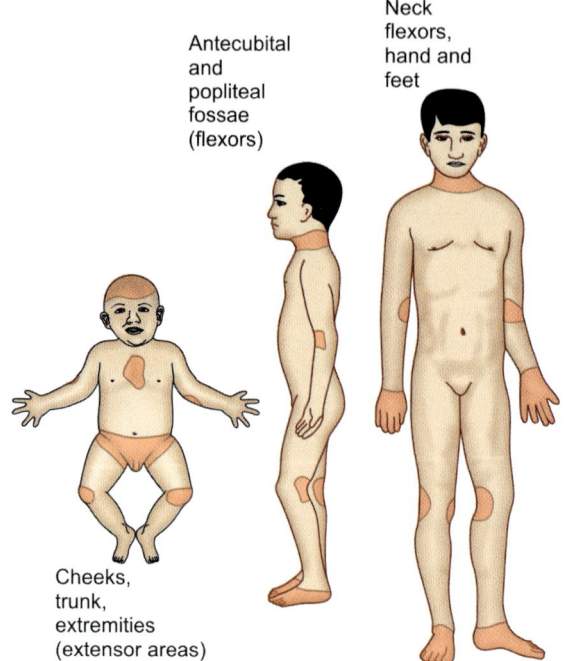

Fig. 8.2: Distribution of atopic eczema across various ages

Infantile Phase (Birth to 2 Years)

The age of onset is usually between the age of 2 and 6 months, but usually not until after 2 months. Eczema in infancy usually begins as erythema and scaling of the cheeks (Figs 8.3a and b).

The eruption may extend to the scalp, neck, forehead, wrists, extensor extremities, and buttocks (Fig. 8.4). The diaper area is usually spared. There may be significant exudate; secondary effects from scratching, rubbing, and infection include crusts, infiltration, and pustules, respectively. Worsening of AD is often observed in infants after immunizations and viral infections. Partial remission may occur during the summer, with relapse in winter.

Childhood Atopic Dermatitis (2–12 Years)

During childhood, lesions tend to be less exudative. The classic locations are the antecubital and popliteal fossae, flexor wrists, eyelids, face, and around the neck. Scratching induces lichenification

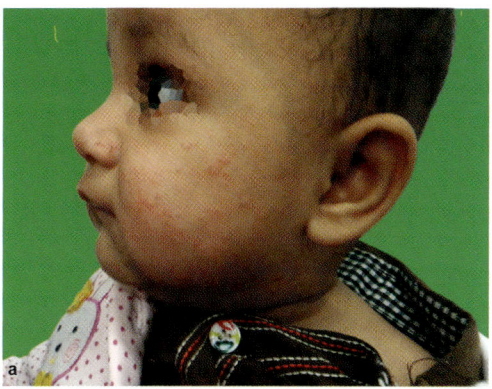

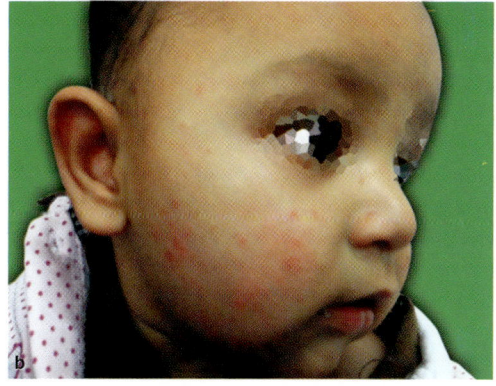

Figs 8.3a and b: Eczematous papules on the cheek in a child will AD

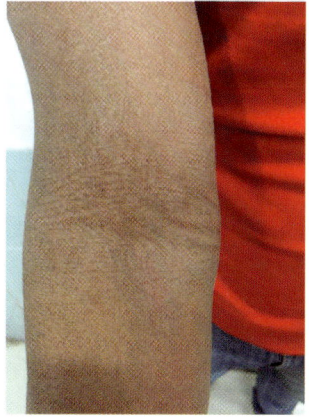

Fig. 8.4: Involvement of flexures in an adult case of AD

and may lead to secondary infection. A vicious cycle may be established, the itch-scratch cycle, as pruritus leads to scratching, and scratching causes secondary changes that in themselves cause itching. Severe AD involving a large percentage of the body surface area can be associated with growth retardation. Restriction diets and steroid use may exacerbate growth impairment.

Atopic Dermatitis in Adolescents and Adults

AD often subsides as the patient grows older, leaving an adult with dry skin that is prone to itching and inflammation when exposed to exogenous irritants. Chronic hand eczema may be the primary manifestation of many adults with AD. AD may begin after age of 18 years in only 6–14% of patients diagnosed with AD. In adolescents, the eruption often involves the classic antecubital and popliteal fossae (Figs 8.5 and 8.6), front and sides of the neck, forehead, and area around the eyes. In older adults, the distribution is generally less characteristic, and localized dermatitis may be the predominant feature, especially hand, nipple, or eyelid eczema. In elderly, like infants, extensors are more commonly involved.

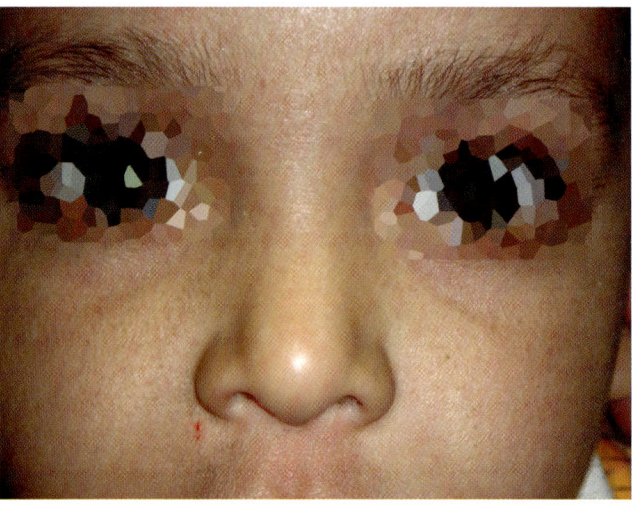

Fig. 8.5: A case of AD with periorbital erythema consequent to frequent rubbing by the patient

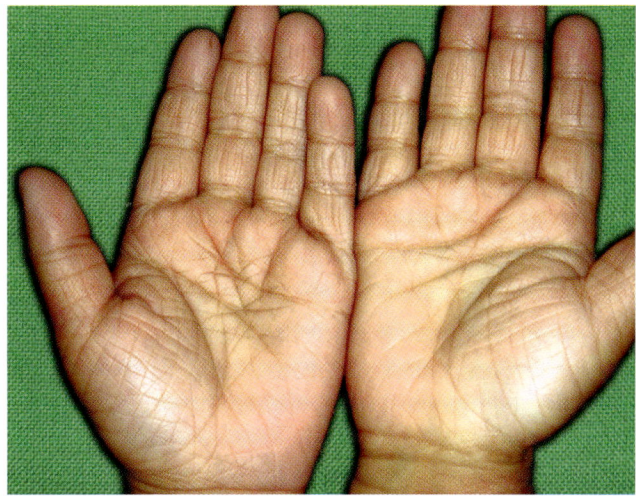

Fig. 8.6: Hyperlinear palms in a case of AD

Regional Variants and Associated Features

Several regional variants of AD can occur in isolation or together with the classic age-related patterns of involvement described above.

Face is a frequent site for various associated findings in AD either alone or in association with classical features of AD.

Eczema of the lips is common in AD patients, especially during the winter. It is characterized by dryness ("chapping") of the vermilion lips, sometimes with peeling and fissuring, and may be associated with angular cheilitis. Patients try to moisten their lips by licking, which in turn, may irritate the skin around the mouth, resulting in so-called **lip-licker's eczema**.

A linear transverse fold just below the edge of the lower eyelids, known as the **Dennie-Morgan fold**, is widely believed to be indicative of AD.

In atopic patients with **eyelid dermatitis**, increased folds and darkening under the eyes (allergic shiners) is common.

Eyelid eczema along with lichenification of periorbital skin may be seen in AD patients (Fig. 8.5).

The less involved skin of atopic patients is frequently dry and slightly erythematous and may be scaly.

Juvenile plantar dermatosis presents with erythema, scale and fissuring on the balls of the feet and plantar aspect of the toes in children with AD, especially during the winter.

Frictional lichenoid eruption has a predilection for atopic children (especially boys) and presents as multiple small, flat topped, pink to skin-colored papules on the elbows and (less often) knees and dorsal hands. It classically occurs in the spring or summer, pruritus is variable, and the histologic findings are nonspecific.

Keratosis pilaris (KP) consists of horny follicular lesions of the outer aspects of the upper arms, legs, cheeks, and buttocks and is often associated with AD. The keratotic papules on the face may be on a red background, a variant of KP called **keratosis pilaris rubra faceii**. KP is often refractory to treatment. Moisturizers alone are only partially beneficial.

Nummular eczema, nipple eczema may be seen in children and adults wth AD.

Hertoghe's sign: Thinning of the lateral eyebrows is sometimes present. This apparently occurs from chronic rubbing caused by pruritus and subclinical dermatitis.

Sometimes patient may just have hyperlinear palms and soles (Fig. 8.6).

Diagnostic Criteria

Several authors and groups have suggested guidelines to assist in establishing the clinical diagnosis of AD.

The criteria proposed by Hanifin and Rajka (Table 8.1) in 1980 are considered to be the 'gold standard' for the clinical diagnosis of AD (Marenholz I et al). UK working party criteria (Table 8.2)

Table 8.1: Hanifin and Rajka criteria

Itchy skin condition (or parental report of scratching or rubbing in a child) Plus
Three or more of the following features: 1. Onset under age of 2 years   2. A history of flexural involvement   3. A history of asthma or hay fever (or a history of atopic disease in siblings and parents if the child is under 4 years).   4. A history of generally dry skin in the last year.   5. Visible flexural dermatitis.

Table 8.2: UK working criteria

Major criteria

Must have three of the following:
1. Pruritus
2. Typical morphology and distribution
   • Flexural lichenification in adults
   • Facial and extensor involvement in infancy
3. Chronic or chronically relapsing dermatitis
4. Personal or family history of atopic disease (e.g. asthma, allergic rhinitis, atopic dermatitis).

Minor criteria

Must also have three of the following:
1. Xerosis
2. Ichthyosis/hyperlinear palms/keratosis pilaris
3. IgE reactivity (immediate skin test reactivity, RAST test positive)
4. Elevated serum IgE
5. Early age of onset
6. Tendency for cutaneous infections (especially *Staphylococcus aureus* and HSV).
7. Tendency to nonspecific hand/foot dermatitis
8. Nipple eczema
9. Cheilitis
10. Recurrent conjunctivitis
11. Dennie-Morgan infraorbital fold
12. Keratoconus
13. Anterior subcapsular cataracts
14. Orbital darkening
15. Facial pallor/facial erythema
16. Pityriasis alba
17. Itch when sweating
18. Intolerance to wool and lipid solvents
19. Perifollicular accentuation
20. Food hypersensitivity
21. Course influenced by environmental and/or emotional factors
22. White dermatographism or delayed blanch to cholinergic agents

RAST: Radioallergosorbent assay; HSV: Herpes simplex virus.

are a simple set of one major and five minor criteria designed for use in population based surveys (Williams HC et al). These criteria are extensively validated and found to be similar to the Hanifin and Rajka criteria in terms of sensitivity and specificity.

Validated scores to assess the severity of AD include the EASI (Eczema Area Scoring Index), SCORAD (SCORing Atopic Dermatitis) and POEM (Patient-Oriented Eczema Measure) [Ricci G et al].

Complications

Ocular Complications

Up to 10% of patients with AD develop cataracts, either anterior or posterior subcapsular. The spectrum of atopic eye disease also includes chronic manifestations such as atopic keratoconjunctivitis (typically in adults) and vernal keratoconjunctivitis (favors children living in warm climates). Atopic keratoconjunctivitis is usually bilateral and can have disabling symptoms that include itching, burning, tearing, and copious mucoid discharge.

Infections

Patients with AD are predisposed to the development of skin infections because of factors including an impaired skin barrier and modified immune milieu. Bacterial and viral infections represent the most common complications of AD. Patient with AD with secondary bacterial infections is frequently associated with weeping and crusting of skin lesions, retro- and infra-auricular and perinasal fissures, folliculitis, and adenopathy.

Eczema herpeticum represents rapid dissemination of a herpes simplex viral infection over the eczematous skin of AD patients. It initially develops as an eruption of vesicles, but affected individuals more often present with numerous monomorphic, punched-out erosions with hemorrhagic crusting. It is often associated with fever, malaise and lymphadenopathy, and complications may include superinfection with *S. aureus* or *S. pyogenes* as well as herpetic keratoconjunctivitis and meningoencephalitis.

Patients with AD are also predisposed to the development of widespread *molluscum contagiosum*.

Superficial fungal infections are also more common in atopic individuals and may contribute to the exacerbation of AD.

Erythroderma

Patients with extensive skin involvement may develop exfoliative dermatitis. This is associated with generalized redness, scaling, weeping, crusting, systemic toxicity, lymphadenopathy, and fever. Although this complication is rare, it is potentially life threatening. In some cases, the withdrawal of systemic glucocorticoids used to control severe AD may be a precipitating factor for exfoliative erythroderma.

DIFFERENTIAL DIAGNOSIS

The differential diagnosis of AD is broad and includes other chronic dermatoses, infections, infestations and malignancies as well as metabolic, genetic (e.g. primary immunodeficiencies) and autoimmune disorders. Depending upon the age of the patient and the clinical presentation, such entities may be considered prior to diagnosing AD, especially when the history, morphology and/or distribution of the skin lesions are atypical.

In children, common conditions that can mimic AD are scabies, seborrheic dermatitis, contact dermatitis and psoriasis.

Rerely immunodeficiency disorders mimic AD such as agammaglobulinemia, Wiskott-Aldrich syndrome, Hyper IgE (Job's syndrome), Omenn's syndrome, Leiner's syndrome.

Other conditions that can mimic AD are acrodermatitis enteropathica, ataxia-telangiectasia, dermatitis herpetiformis, Langerhans cell histiocytosis, Hurler syndrome and phenylketo-nuria.

INVESTIGATION

Laboratory testing is **not** needed in the routine evaluation and treatment of uncomplicated AD. Serum IgE levels are elevated in approximately 70–80% of AD patients. The majority of patients with AD also have peripheral blood eosinophilia.

Classical tests for IgE-mediated hypersensitivity are skin prick test and RAST (radioallergosorbent test for specific IgEs in the blood). The atopy patch test is one of the recently described tests in AD and is preferred for aeroallergen testing.

For food allergies the double-blind placebo controlled food challenge (DBPCFC) is considered to be the gold standard.

Till date there is no gold standard test for confirmation of allergies in patients with AD.

Histopathology is not diagnostic and similar findings are observed in other eczematous dermatoses such as allergic contact dermatitis.

The histology of AD varies with the stage of the lesion, with many of the changes induced by scratching.

TREATMENT

Parental and patient education is very important in the management of AD.

Because AD is a chronic relapsing disease, the classic approach to therapy is targeting acute flares with short-term treatment regimens, i.e. reactive management. Based on recent insights into the underlying skin barrier defect and its relationship to inflammatory processes in the skin and other organs, a proactive approach that includes long-term maintenance therapy is now recommended (Wollenberg A et al).

Multipronged approach that incorporates education about the disease state, skin hydration, pharmacologic therapy, and the identification and elimination of flare factors such as irritants, allergens, infectious agents, and emotional stressors constitutes successful treatment.

Management strategy should be adapted to the severity of the disease. Mild cases are typically controlled by continuous use of emollients and intermittent use of a low-potency topical corticosteroid for flares, moderate AD may also require proactive maintenance with anti-inflammatory agents. In more severe and refractory cases, the use of phototherapy and systemic drugs may be necessary to control the disease.

Elimination of Aggravating Factors

Number of environmental aggravating factors have been identified in AD. Careful history in determining specific aggravating factors and further avoidance of exposure to such triggering factors may help in avoiding exacerbations. Couselling regarding modification of lifestyle may help in avoiding triggers. Some important lifestyle modification measures are detailed in Table 8.3.

Table 8.3: Lifestyle modification measures to avoid trigger factors to AD

Avoiding aeroallergens

1. Frequent wet mopping of floors and surfaces.
2. Avoid pets.
3. Avoid carpets rugs.
4. Plastic covering of matresses.

Clothing

1. Avoid woollen or synthetic clothing.
2. Use cotton clothing which covers exremities.

Food allergens

1. Advise exclusive breastfeeding till 6 months of age.
2. Elimination diets should not be routinely advised unless its confirmed by oral food challenge tests.

Bathing and detergent contact

1. Use of mild soaps preferably syndets with pH around 6.
2. Avoidance of frequent or lengthy bathing.
3. Soap should be applied only to intertriginous sites (groin and axillae).
4. Liberal use of emollients to moist skin after bathing to trap moisture.
5. Topical medications should be applied first to the affected areas of skin, with emollient applied afterwards to the non-affected areas of skin.

Barrier Repair

Critical role of an impaired skin barrier in the pathogenesis of AD underscore the importance of a continuous basic therapy with emollients, even in periods and sites in which the AD is not active.

Ointments (e.g. petrolatum) and water-in-oil creams are more occlusive and tend to cause less burning and stinging than oil-in-water creams and lotions. However, the greasiness of an ointment is not acceptable to all patients.

Emollients should be applied twice daily to the entire cutaneous surface. Emollients containing particular combinations of lipids that are normally present in the stratum corneum (e.g. cholesterol, fatty acids, ceramides) may optimize barrier repair. Potentially allergy-provoking ingredients such as perfumes, lanolin and herbal extracts should be avoided.

Oral Antihistamines

Antihistamines are frequently used but pruritus of AD is notoriously resistant to antihistamines especially nonsedating ones. If prescribed, sedating antihistamines are used nightly to break "itch scratch cycle" (not "as needed"). Diphenhydramine, hydroxyzine, and doxepin can all be efficacious.

Topical Anti-inflammatory Drugs

Topical Steroids

Topical steroids are used in the management of AD in both adults and children and are the mainstay of anti-inflammatory therapy. They suppress production of several transcription factors, which leads not only to reduced expression of proinflammatory cytokines but also to inhibition of cell growth and decreased synthesis of collagen and other structural proteins (explaining side effects such as skin atrophy. They are typically introduced into the treatment regimen after failure of lesions to respond to good skin care and regular use of moisturizers alone. In most body sites, once-daily application of a corticosteroid is almost as effective as more frequent applications, at lower cost and with less systemic absorption. In infants, low-potency steroid ointments, such as hydrocortisone, desonide are preferred. In older children and adults, medium-potency steroids such as fluicasone, mometasone are often used, except on the face, where milder steroids or calcineurin inhibitors are preferred. Proactive, intermittent use of TCS as maintenance therapy (2–3 times per week) on areas that commonly flare is recommended to help prevent relapses while reducing the need for topical corticosteroids, and is more effective than the use of emollients alone.

If an atopic patient worsens or fails to improve after the use of topical steroids and moisturizers, the possibility of allergic contact dermatitis to a preservative or the corticosteroids must be considered. The incidence of reported side effects from TCS use is low; however, long term use may cause potential complications which include purpura, telangiectasia, striae, focal hypertrichosis, and acneiform or rosacea-like eruptions. Many of these side effects will resolve after discontinuing TCS use, but may take months.

Topical Calcineurin Inhibitors

US Food and Drug Administration (FDA) for the treatment of AD: tacrolimus 0.03% and 0.1% ointment (for "moderate to severe" disease) and pimecrolimus 1% cream (for "mild to moderate" disease). These agents suppress T cell activation and modulate the secretion of cytokines and other proinflammatory mediators. Their efficacy in the treatment of AD has been proven in clinical trials in adults and children at least 2 years of age (and, for pimecrolimus, infants ages 3–23 months, although it is not approved for this group).

The major side effect of both medications is burning at the site of application; they are not associated with cutaneous atrophy. In 2006, the FDA introduced black box warnings for both drugs concerning a theoretical cancer risk.

Topical calcineurin inhibitors are particularly useful on the eyelids and face, in areas prone to steroid atrophy, when steroid allergy is a consideration, or when systemic steroid absorption is a concern.

Recent randomized controlled studies have shown that the proactive application of tacrolimus ointment (e.g. twice weekly as maintenance) can prevent flares of AD without increasing the overall amount of medication used.

Treatment of Bacterial Infections

Topical or oral antibiotics should be reserved for cases with frank evidence of secondary infection, which may worsen eczema through action of superantigens.

Bleach bathes which reduce staphylococcal colonization have rapidly become a mainstay in AD patients. Tepid bath with ¼ cup of standard household bleach (6%) diluted in 20 gallons of water used twice a week dramaticsally improves AD on the trunk and extremities, but less so on the face.

Intranasal application of mupirocin is beneficial in reducing nasal carriage of staphylococci.

Phototherapy

All forms of phototherapy like PUVA, narrowband UV B, broadband UV B, UVA1 are effective in treatment of AD and are mainly used for long-term maintenance treatment, along with topicals.

NBUVB is preferable to PUVA especially in children due to its better tolerability and safety profile.

UVB mainly acts by inhibiting antigen presentation by langerhans cells, T cell activation and cytokine production by keratinocytes.

Systemic Treatment

Systemic anti-inflammatory treatment should be restricted to severe, refractory cases of AD that do not respond adequately to intensive topical therapy. Of note, no systemic medications besides corticosteroids have been FDA-approved for treatment of AD.

In general, *systemic corticosteroids* should be used only to control acute exacerbations. In patients requiring systemic steroid therapy, short courses (≤3weeks) are preferred. If repeated or prolonged courses of systemic corticosteroids are required to control the AD, phototherapy or a steroid-sparing agent should be considered. Systemic steroids are not a preferred agent in children with AD due to their side effect profile and rebound flare on withdrawal.

Cyclosporin A is one of the most commonly used systemic agents for AD as it is shown to be safe and effective in both children and adults, although probably tolerated better in children. Oral cyclosporin 3–5 mg/kg/day typically leads to rapid improvement of skin disease and associated pruritus in patients with AD, and its efficacy has been established in randomized controlled trials.

It is very useful to gain rapid control of severe AD. Potential long-term side effects, especially nephrotoxicity, require careful monitoring, with attempts to transition the patient to a potentially less toxic agent when possible.

Azathioprine can be an effective treatment for moderate to severe AD in children and adults, with modest benefit. It is used in dose of 2.5–3.5 mg/kg/day along with other treatment modalities simultaneously.

Other immunosuppressive agents that can be used are *mycophenolate* mofetil and *methotrexate*.

TREATMENT PLAN

As all patients of atopic dermatitis are different an individualized approach is needed depending on the severity of AD, thus in mild cases topical emollients and mild steroids may suffice, but this may not apply to all cases of AD. Another treatment approach is given below.

This treatment plan consists of two steps

a. A short "acute" phase of treatment (1 to 2 weeks), the purpose of which is to obtain the fullest clinical remission possible as quickly as possible. This phase is based on the once a day usage of a topical steroid that is suitable in terms of potency and pharmaceutical form for the patient according to their age and lesion sites. The treatment is stopped *without* gradual tapering off as soon as erythema and pruritus disappear. There is no maximum recommended amount during acute phase treatment. If the acute phase treatment is as effective as expected, maintenance treatment can begin. It will be assessed in terms of efficacy and tolerability after 6 to 8 weeks. If it is not effective, compliance may be a issue (ask questions, check whether there is a fear of steroids, count the number of tubes used since the last appointment). If adherence is satisfactory, the second line treatment must be started, including potent steroids, phototherapy or systemic agents. This method is called the *early reactive treatment*. This is indicated in cases of AD with flare-ups that are spaced several weeks apart.

b. A "*maintenance*" phase, the purpose of which is to maintain remission in the long-term. This phase consists of:

   • Daily usage of emollients;

   • Usage of a topical steroid or even topical tacrolimus following one of two different regimens. Topical steroids are often prescribed as a first line treatment for maintenance. Topical tacrolimus is offered as a second line treatment where topical steroids have failed or as a first line treatment if there is a contraindication to topical steroids or in certain high-risk sites (especially the face).

     – This approach is called *proactive treatment*. This is indicated in forms with flare-ups that follow on quickly one after another or when symptoms are permanent (this means when lesions reappear as soon as anti-inflammatory treatment is stopped). It entails using anti-inflammatory treatment routinely (even in the absence of lesions) on the areas that are usually affected, 2 to 3 times a week over a long period of time (several weeks or even months). This method leads to a clear reduction in the number of flare-ups in the medium term and a decrease in the amount of anti-inflammatory used when compared to a standard reactive treatment regimen. If a flare-up develops during maintenance treatment, the same principles as for the acute phase treatment are applicable while the flare-up is being treated.

Bibliography

1. Asher MI, Montefort S, Bjorksten B, et al. Worldwide time trends in the prevalence of symptoms of asthma, allergic rhinoconjunctivitis, and eczema in childhood: ISAAC Phases One and Three repeat multicountry crosssectional surveys. Lancet 2006;368:733–43.

2. Barker JN, Palmer CN, Zhao Y, Liao H, Hull PR, Lee SP, Allen MH, Meggitt SJ, Reynolds NJ, Trembath RC, McLean WH. Null mutations in the filaggrin gene (FLG) determine major susceptibility to early-onset atopic dermatitis that persists into adulthood. J Invest Dermatol 2007 Mar;127(3):564–7. Epub 2006 Sep 21.

3. Bratton DL, et al Granulocyte macrophage colony-stimulating factor contributes to enhanced monocyte survival in chronic atopic dermatitis. J Clin Invest 1995;95:211.

4. Bunikowski R, Mielke M, Skarabis H, et al. Prevalence and role of serum IgE antibodies to the *Staphylococcus aureus*-derived superantigens SEA and SEB in children with atopic dermatitis. J Allergy Clin Immunol 1999; 103:119–24.

5. Cho SH, Strickland I, Boguniewicz M, Leung DY: Fibronectin and fibrinogen contribute to the enhanced binding of *Staphylococcus aureus* to atopic skin. J Allergy Clin Immunol 2001 Aug;108(2):269–74.

6. DaVeiga SP. Epidemiology of atopic dermatitis: a review. Allergy Asthma Proc 2012 May-Jun;33(3):227–34. doi: 10.2500/aap 2012.33. 3569.

7. Eichenfield LF, Ellis CN, Mancini AJ, Paller AS, Simpson EL. Atopic dermatitis: epidemiology and pathogenesis update. Semin Cutan Med Surg. 2012 Sep;31(3 Suppl):S3–5. doi: 10.1016/j.sder.2012.07.002.

8. Elias PM, Hatano Y, Williams ML. Basis for the barrier abnormality in atopic dermatitis: outside-inside-outside pathogenic mechanisms. J Allergy Clin Immunol 2008 Jun;121(6):1337-43. doi: 10.1016/j.jaci.2008. 01.022. Epub 2008 Mar 7.

9. Kanwar AJ, De D. Epidemiology and clinical features of atopic dermatitis in India. Indian J Dermatol 2011;56:471–5.

10. Marenholz I, Kerscher T, Bauerfeind A, Esparza-Gordillo J, Nickel R, Keil T, Lau S, Rohde K, Wahn U, Lee YA. An interaction between

filaggrin mutations and early food sensitization improves the prediction of childhood asthma. J Allergy Clin Immunol 2009 Apr;123(4):911-6. doi: 10.1016/j.jaci.2009.01.051.

11. Ricci G, Dondi A, Patrizi A. Useful tools for the management of atopic dermatitis. Am J Clin Dermatol 2009;10:287–300.

12. Strachan DP. Hay fever, hygiene, and household size. BMJ 1989;299:1259.

13. Superantigens in atopic dermatitis: implications for future therapeutic strategies. Am J Clin Dermatol 2006;7:273–9.

14. Toda M, et al: Polarized in vivo expression of IL-11 and IL-17 between acute and chronic skin lesions. J Allergy Clin Immunol 2003;111:875.

15. Williams HC. Clinical practice. Atopic dermatitis. N Engl J Med 2005;352:2314–24.

16. Williams HC, Burney PG, Hay RJ, Archer CB, Shipley MJ, Hunter JJ, Bingham EA, Finlay AY, Pembroke AC, Graham-Brown RA, et al. The U.K. Working Party's Diagnostic Criteria for Atopic Dermatitis. I. Derivation of a minimum set of discriminators for atopic dermatitis. Br J Dermatol 1994 Sep;131(3):383–96.

17. Wollenberg A, Bieber T. Proactive therapy of atopic dermatitis—an emerging concept. Allergy 2009;64:276–8.

Seborrheic Eczema

INTRODUCTION

Seborrheic eczema or seborrheic dermatitis (SD) is a common dermatitis that affects both adults and infants. It is estimated to affect all ethnic groups and both genders, and can adversely affect the quality of life (Szepietowski JC et al, Manapajon A et al). There are several epidemiologic studies on SD looking at the prevalence and gender predilection in different populations (Palamaras et al). The prevalence for adult SD ranges from 2.35% in Scotland (Ratzer), 4.05% in Greece (Palamaras et al), 4.3% in Iran (Baghestani et al), 6.9% in Australia (Plunkett et al) and 7% in Singapore (Goh et al). Infantile SD has a prevalence of 2.5% in Greece (Palamaras et al), 3.1% in Kuwait (Nanda et al), 4.3% in Turkey (Tamer et al) and 11.3% in India (Sardana et al).

A study conducted in an Indian pediatric population noted 13.42% of children below 5 years were affected by SD. This involved infants predominantly and was worse during winter (Banerjee S et al). Another study from India looking at scalp dermatoses in adults visiting a tertiary referral center reported 18.7% of their cohort with scalp SD (Pillai et al).

ETIOLOGY AND PREDISPOSING FACTORS

Seborrheic dermatitis is more commonly seen in adult patients with Parkinson's disease (Binder RL et al), as well as in immuno-compromised states induced by the human immunodeficiency virus (HIV) (Mathes BM et al). In temperate climates, SD can be worse in the winter months. It is also reported to be aggravated by hot climate (Manapajon A et al). Other diseases that have been reported to occur with SD include chronic alcoholic pancreatitis (Barba A et al), hepatitis C infections (Cribier B et al), malignancies (Clift DC), Down syndrome (Ercis M et al), Hailey Hailey disease (Marren P et al) and cardiofaciocutaneous syndromes syndromes (Gross-Tsur V et al). Drug related SD is less commonly seen but should be suspected in patients who are exposed to drugs including erlotinib or sorafenib, recombinant interleukin-2, psoralen plus ultraviolet A light and isotretinoin (Naldi L et al).

The pathogenesis of SD is postulated to arise from an interaction between yeasts from the Malassezia genus with the immune system (Hay RJ). Metabolites from the Malassezia yeasts such as malassezin and indole-3-carbaldehyde interacts with the aryl hydrocarbon receptor and modulates immune responses to the Malassezia yeasts (Gaitanis G et al). The role of Malassezia yeasts is shown indirectly by the resolution of SD after treatment with antifungal agents (Shuster S). In addition, alterations in sebum production (Ostlere et al, Henderson et al) and androgenic hormonal influence is postulated to play a role as well.

CLINICAL PHENOTYPES

Infantile SD is often a self-limited condition that presents in the 2nd to 10th week of life, peaks at 3 months and resolves by 5 to 6 months. In patients with a family history of atopy, a significant portion (30–40%) goes on to develop atopic dermatitis (Alexopoulos A et al). Most infants with SD have mild disease (dandruff, cradle cap, involvement of the eyebrows, paranasal areas and intertriginous areas). The differential diagnoses to consider include infantile atopic dermatitis, infantile psoriasis, neonatal acne, Langerhans' cell histiocytosis, food allergies manifesting as worsening dermatitis and inherited or acquired zinc deficiency.

In rare instances when infants present with SD-like erythroderma and failure to thrive, one has to consider other differential diagnoses including genodermatoses, primary immune deficiency (Leiner's disease), metabolic disease or infection (Fraitag S et al). These infants require specialized investigations and management by dermatologists.

Adult SD affects areas with high sebaceous gland activity. Mild SD on the scalp can present with dandruff. In severe cases of scalp SD, thick scales with matted hairs typical of pityriasis amiantacea can occur (Fig. 9.1). On the *face*, SD typically presents with persistent scaly, thin pink papules and plaques on the medial aspects of the eyebrows, nasolabial folds and periauricular areas and sometimes with overlying yellowish oily scales (Fig. 9.2). On the *trunk* (presternal and interscapular areas), SD presents with thin pink papules and plaques with fine scaling in a petaloid (described as circinate patches with a light-red scaling area in the center and darker red papules at their margin, (Fig. 9.3) or pityriasiform pattern. SD may also affect the axilla, submammary area, umbilicus and anogenital area. Other dermatological conditions that can mimic SD include psoriasis, eczema, contact dermatitis and superficial fungal infections. In patients with HIV infection, SD is often more inflammatory and extensively distributed.

In rare instances, genodermatoses (Darier's disease and Hailey Hailey disease), immunobullous disease (pemphigus foliaceus) and infections (secondary syphilis) can mimic adult SD on the trunk and flexures while acute lupus and rosacea can mimic adult facial SD. Patients should be assessed by a dermatologist if atypical features (photosensitivity, erosive lesions, persistent disease despite adequate treatment) are present.

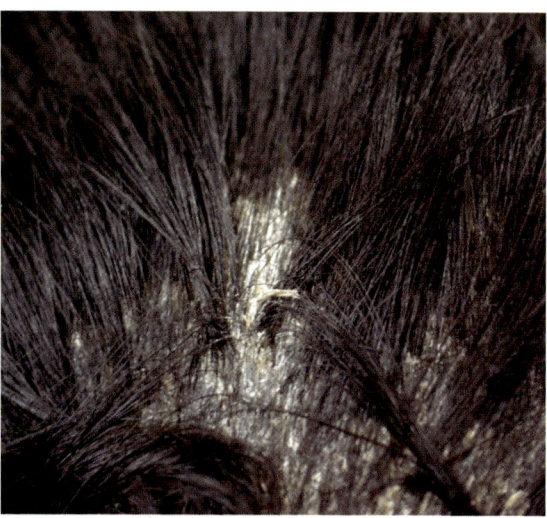

Fig. 9.1: Seborrheic dermatitis of the scalp in a 15-year-old male showing thick adherent scales typical of pityriasis amiantacea

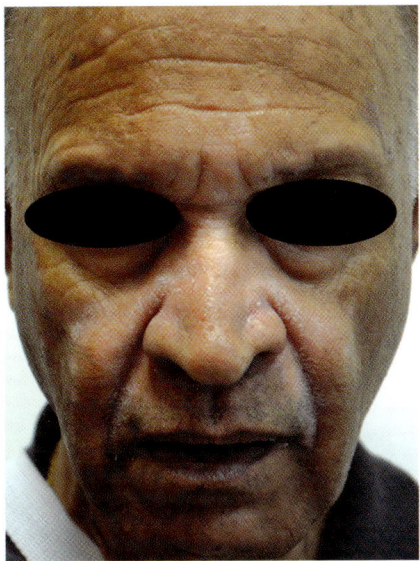

Fig. 9.2: Seborrheic dermatitis affecting the nasolabial folds and medial corners of the eyebrows

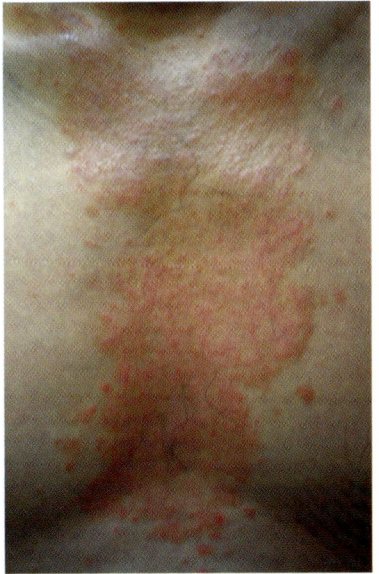

Fig. 9.3: Seborrheic dermatitis affecting the presternal area in a petaloid pattern

INVESTIGATIONS

In infants presenting with mild SD, the diagnosis is clinical and further investigations are not necessary. However, when infants present with SD and other atypical features (e.g. poor response to treatment, recurrent severe flares, failure to thrive), a referral to a dermatologist is recommended for further evaluation.

The diagnosis of SD is based on clinical findings in adults and further investigations are not necessary if the clinical presentation is typical. In cases where the diagnosis of SD is in doubt, skin biopsy for histological examination can be useful to differentiate SD from other skin disorders.

TREATMENT

Many treatment options are available to control SD. These treatments target the various pathogenic factors that cause SD, including topical and oral antifungal medication, nonsteroidal cream with antifungal and anti-inflammatory properties, topical steroids and topical calcineurin inhibitors. The treatment of SD should be tailored to the location and severity of SD in the individual patients, bearing in mind that SD is a chronic condition with frequent recurrence after treatment in adults, while it is often self-limiting in mild cases of infantile SD.

Published peer-reviewed guidelines for the treatment of adult SD are available (Hald M et al, Naldi et al). Adults with *mild to moderate* scalp SD (mild to moderate scaling, itching with a few papules) can benefit from topical shampoos with antifungal effects (e.g. shampoos containing 2% ketoconazole. 1% ciclopirox, 2.5% selenium sulfide, 1–2% zinc pyrithione, 1–2% coal tar). These should be applied 2 to 3 times weekly for 3 to 4 weeks. *For severe scalp* SD (generalized scaling and erythema with severe itching), a topical steroid scalp lotion (e.g. 0.1% betamethasone valerate) applied 1 to 2 times daily for 1 to 2 weeks can be used in addition to the antifungal shampoo to achieve disease control.

Adults with *mild to moderate facial and truncal SD* can be treated with topical antifungal creams twice daily (e.g. 2% ketoconazole, 1% ciclopirox). Topical steroid creams of the appropriate potency for the site of SD can be added to achieve rapid control of SD. In *moderate to severe cases of adult SD*, topical steroids are often required to achieve control (Fig. 9.4). Usage of topical steroids should be limited to not more than 1–2 weeks. Topical calcineurin inhibitors (1% pimecrolimus, 0.1% and 0.03% tacrolimus ointment) can be used off label as a steroid sparing alternative for moderate to severe adult SD, but its use may be hampered by local irritation and cost. A nonsteroidal medical device cream with antifungal properties (Sebclair™, A Menarini) has been shown to be effective in *mild to moderate adult SD* (Veraldi S et al, Elewski B). This may be considered for use as monotherapy and maintenance therapy.

Infantile SD should be managed more conservatively as the condition is often mild and self-limiting. Simple measures such as regular washing of the scalp with a mild baby shampoo and gentle combing to loosen scales is often enough to treat mild cradle cap. Topical emollients (olive oil, white petrolatum) can be added as an adjunct to soften and loosen adherent scales on the scalp. Topical medicated shampoos (2% ketoconazole, cetrimide, coal tar) on alternate days can be used for added effect on cradle cap. A nonsteroidal cream with anti-inflammatory and antifungal properties (Sebclair™, A Menarini) has been shown to be effective in the treatment of mild to moderate cradle cap (David E et al).

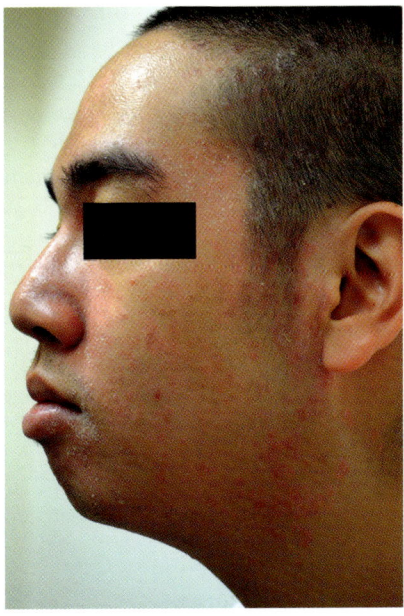

Fig. 9.4: Severe seborrheic dermatitis involving the scalp and face

Mild topical steroids (e.g. 1% hydrocortisone cream applied sparingly over affected areas daily to every other day) and topical antifungal creams (ketoconazole 2% cream daily to every other day) can be used for infantile SD on the skin folds over 2 to 4 weeks to achieve control (Cohen S). There are concerns of systemic absorption with topical steroids, leading to adrenal suppression in infants (Turpeinen M et al), while no systemic absorption for topical ketoconazole was found when it was used to treat infantile SD (Taieb A et al).

Patients with severe generalized adult or infantile SD, SD with atypical features or those that fail to achieve disease control after 2 to 4 weeks of therapy should be assessed and managed by a specialized dermatologist.

Bibliography

1. Alexopoulos A, Kakourou T, Orfanou I, Xaidara A, Chrousos G. Retrospective analysis of the relationship between infantile seborrheic dermatitis and atopic dermatitis. Pediatr Dermatol 2014;31:125–30.

2. Baghestani S, Zare S, Mahboobi AA. Skin disease patterns in Hormozgan, Iran. Int J Dermatol 2005; 44: 641–645.

3. Banerjee S, Gangopadhyay DN, Jana S, Chanda M.Seasonal variation in pediatric dermatoses.Indian J Dermatol 2010;55:44–6.

4. Barba A, Piubello W, Vantini I, et al. Skin lesions in chronic alcoholic pancreatitis. Dermatologica 1982;164:322–326.

5. Binder RL, Jonelis FJ. Seborrheic dermatitis in neuroleptic induced parkinsonism. Arch Dermatol 1983;119:473–475.

6. Clift DC, Dodd JH, Kirby JD, et al. Seborrheic dermatitis and malignancy. An investigation of the skin flora. Acta Derm Venereol 1988;68:48–52.

7. Cohen S.Should we treat infantile seborrhoeic dermatitis with topical antifungals or topical steroids? Arch Dis Child 2004;89:288–9.

8. Cribier B, Samain F, Vetter D, et al. Systematic cutaneous examination in hepatitis C virus infected patients. Acta Derm Venereol 1992;72:454–455.

9. David E, Tanuos H, Sullivan T, Yan A, Kircik LH. A double-blind, placebo-controlled pilot study to estimate the efficacy and tolerability of a nonsteroidal cream for the treatment of cradle cap (seborrheic dermatitis). J Drugs Dermatol 2013;12:448–52.

10. Elewski B.An investigator-blind, randomized, 4-week, parallel-group, multicenter pilot study to compare the safety and efficacy of

a nonsteroidal cream (Promiseb Topical Cream) and desonide cream 0.05% in the twice-daily treatment of mild to moderate seborrheic dermatitis of the face. Clin Dermatol 2009;27(6 Suppl):S48–53.

11. Ercis M, Balci S, Atakan N. Dermatological manifestations of 71 Down syndrome children admitted to a clinical genetics unit. Clin Genet 1996;50:317–320.

12. Fraitag S, Bodemer C. Neonatal erythroderma. Curr Opin Pediatr 2010; 22 :438–44.

13. Gaitanis G, Magiatis P, Stathopoulou K, et al. AhR ligands, malassezin, and indolo 3, 2-b carbazole are selectively produced by *Malassezia furfur* strains isolated from seborrheic dermatitis. J Invest Dermatol 2008; 128:1620–5.

14. Goh CL, Akarapanth R. Epidemiology of skin disease among children in a referral skin clinic in Singapore. Pediatr Dermatol 1994;11:125–128.

15. Gross-Tsur V, Gross-Kieselstein E, Amir N. Cardio-faciocutaneous syndrome: neurological manifestations. Clin Genet 1990;38:382–386.

16. Hald M, Arendrup MC, Svejgaard EL, Lindskov R, Foged EK, Saunte DM; Danish Society of Dermatology.Evidence-based Danish guidelines for the treatment of Malassezia-related skin diseases.Acta Derm Venereol 2015;95:12–9.

17. Hay RJ. Malassezia, dandruff and seborrhoeic dermatitis: an overview. Br J Dermatol 2011;165 Suppl 2:2–8.

18. Henderson CA, Taylor J, Cunliffe WJ. Sebum excretion rates in mothers and neonates. Br J Dermatol 2000;142:110–111.

19. Manapajon A, Kanokvalai K, Sukhum J. Clinical characteristics and quality of life of seborrheic dermatitis patients in a tropical country. Indian J Dermatology 2015; 60:519.

20. Marren P, Burge S. Seborrhoeic dermatitis of the scalp—a manifestation of Hailey?Hailey disease in a predisposed individual. Br J Dermatol 1992;126:294–296.

21. Mathes BM, Douglass MC. Seborrheic dermatitis in patients with acquired immunodeficiency syndrome. J Am Acad Dermatol 1985;13: 947–951.

22. Naldi L, Rebora A.Clinical practice. Seborrheic dermatitis.N Engl J Med. 2009;360:387–96.

23. Nanda A, Al-Hasawi F, Alsaleh QA. A prospective survey of pediatric dermatology clinic patients in Kuwait: an analysis of 10,000 cases. Pediatr Dermatol 1999; 16: 6–11.

24. Ostlere LS, Taylor CR, Harris DW, et al. Skin surface lipids in HIV positive patients with and without seborrheic dermatitis. Int J Dermatol 1996;35:276–9.

25. Palamaras I, Kyriakis KP, Stavrianeas NG. Seborrheic dermatitis: lifetime detection rates. J Eur Acad Dermatol Venereol 2012;26:524–6.

26. Pillai J, Okade R. A clinical spectrum of scalp dermatoses in adults presenting to a tertiary referral care centre. Int J Biol Med Res 2014;5:4434–4439.

27. Plunkett A, Merlin K, Gill D, Zuo Y, Jolley D, Marks R. The frequencyof common nonmalignant skin conditions in adults in central Victoria, Australia. Int J Dermatol 1999; 38: 901–908.

28. Ratzer MA. The incidence of skin diseases in the West of Scotland.Br J Dermatol 1969;81:456–461.

29. Sardana K, Mahajan S, Sarkar R, et al. The spectrum of skin disease among Indian children. Pediatr Dermatol 2009;26:6–13.

30. Shuster S. The aetiology of dandruff and the mode of action of therapeutic agents. Br J Dermatol 1984;111:235–42.

31. Szepietowski JC, Reich A, Weso?owska-Szepietowska E, Baran E. National Quality of Life in Dermatology Group. Quality of life in patients suffering from seborrheic dermatitis: influence of age, gender and education level.Mycoses. 2009;52:357–63.

32. Taieb A, Legrain V, Palmier C, et al. Topical ketoconazole for infantile seborrhoeic dermatitis. Dermatologica 1990;181:26–32.

33. Tamer E, Ilhan MN, Polat M, Lenk N, Alli N. Prevalence of skin diseases among pediatric patients in Turkey. J Dermatol 2008; 35: 413–418.

34. Turpeinen M, Salo OP, Leisti S. Effect of percutaneous absorption of hydrocortisone on adrenocortical responsiveness in infants with severe skin disease. Br J Dermatol 1986;115:475–484.

35. Veraldi S, Menter A, Innocenti M.Treatment of mild to moderate seborrhoeic dermatitis with MAS064D (Sebclair), a novel topical medical device: results of a pilot, randomized, double-blind, controlled trial.J Eur Acad Dermatol Venereol 2008;22:290–6.

10

Asteatotic Eczema

This pruritic dermatitis is most commonly located in the lower extremities of elderly individuals, but may present in other parts of the body as well.

CLINICAL FEATURES

The affected areas appear dry, with fine scales and cracks that can coalesce in a perpendicular fashion, resembling cracks in porcelain (Fig. 10.1) or cement. The term eczema craquelé is appropriately used to describe this pattern. Though seen on the lower limb, this can involve the trunk also in severe cases. Scratching or treatment

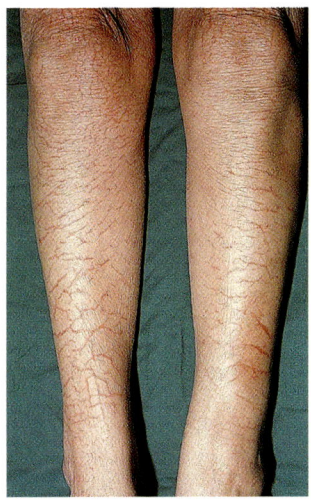

Fig. 10.1: Xerosis with cracked skin (eczema craquelé)

with drying lotions such as calamine *aggravates* the eczematous inflammation and leads to infection with accumulation of crusts and purulent material.

It is most commonly associated with vigorous cleaning and rubbing, hot baths, and a history of xerosis. In India, it is also seen in areas where "hard water " is used for bathing purposes. Patients with an atopic diathesis are more likely to develop this distinctive pattern.

PATHOGENESIS

It is thought to occur more commonly in the elderly population in the setting of xerosis, secondary to a decrease in sebaceous and sweat gland activity, in addition to epidermal water loss in the barrier. Frequent bathing with soap, especially during the winter, is a common factor in the elderly. The combination of *hot water*, *harsh soaps* and *hard water* lead to a increase in this condition. Fundamentally, most asteatotic eczema represents a barrier defect. Spongiotic change is secondary. Some cases represent mild forms of nummular eczema.

TREATMENT

Gentle cleaning with emollients and lukewarm water is recommended. In mild cases the treatment is like for cases of subacute eczema (see above), rarely are compresses required, which is the therapy for acute eczema.

Topical corticosteroids can be considered if there is an inflammatory component. In addition, 12% ammonium lactate lotion may help soften dry skin, but patients should be cautioned that it occasionally stings and irritates fissured areas. The use of oral steroids should be avoided as the disease flares within 1 or 2 days once they are discontinued.

Bibliography

1. Eczema, in. Sardana k, Mahajan S, Garg VK. Diagnosis and Management of Skin Disorders: An Evidence-Based Approach, 1/ e.: Lippincott Williams and Wilkins, 2012 (reprint 2015).
2. Fast Facts: Eczema and Contact Dermatitis By John Berth-Jones, Eunice Tan and Howard I Malbach Published 2004.
3. Thieme Clinical Companions Dermatology. Sterry, Dermatology© 2006 Thieme.

11

Discoid Eczema

Discoid eczema (also known as "Numular dermatitis") is one of the many forms of dermatitis. It is also known as **discoid dermatitis**. The name comes from the Latin word "nummus," which means" coin. It is characterized by round or oval coin shaped itchy lesions over the extensor surfaces of the upper extremities. It was first described in the mid 1800s by Marie Guillaume Alphonse Devergie and classically presents in younger to middle-aged patients (Devergie M). It is to be distinguished from an irregular patchy form of eczema in which the lesions do not have recognizable, clear margins.

ETIOLOGY

The etiology of nummular eczema is multifactorial, involving environmental, allergic, emotional, and nutritional factors. It can occur in any season, but due to increased use of hot water, soaps, and detergents, it is most frequent in the colder months and was once termed "winter eczema" for this reason. It is associated with dryness of the skin, which may allow epidermal breach and permeation of allergens (Aoyama H). Severe, generalized nummular eczema has been reported in association with interferon and ribavirin therapy for hepatitis C and tumor necrosis factor inhibitors (Shen Y).

Some have stressed the role of infection. As in other forms of eczema, heavy colonization of the lesions by staphylococci may increase their severity, even in the absence of clinical evidence of infection (Wachs GN). However, allergic sensitivity to staphylococci or micrococci may be responsible at least for secondary dissemination.

CLINICAL FEATURES

Men usually get nummular eczema late in their life while women get it at a younger age. Location is important to the diagnosis and most commonly involves the dorsa of the hands, extensor surfaces of the forearms, upper arms, legs, thighs, and feet. The lesions start as solid plaques that enlarge and develop a peripheral papulovesicular border (Fig. 11.1). There is often associated pruritis, but this varies greatly, with some patients complaining of almost constant itching and others noticing severe pruritis only at the time of initial outbreak of new lesions.

It may be convenient to recognize the following patterns:
1. Discoid eczema of the *hands and forearms*
2. Discoid eczema of the *limbs and trunk*
3. *Dry* discoid eczema.

Discoid eczema of the hands is not a uncommon form of irritant occupational dermatitis, but may also occur in housewives or secretaries in whom the provoking factors are less clear. An atopic history appears to be more frequent in young women with discoid hand eczema than in other forms of the disease.

The more usual form of discoid eczema affects the limbs (Fig. 11.1) and trunk. It appears to be particularly prevalent among managerial or professional classes. It is also seen in elderly people, often with dry skin exacerbated by low humidity, central heating, car heating, etc.

Dry discoid eczema is an uncommon variant, consisting of multiple, dry, scaly, round or oval discs on the arms or legs (Fig. 11.2), but also with scattered microvesicles on an erythematous base on the palms and soles.

Course: Nummular dermatitis often waxes and wanes with winter; cold or dry climates or swings in temperature may be exacerbating factors. It may improve with sun or humidity exposure or with moisturizer use. Occasionally it may worsen with heat or humidity. New nummular dermatitis lesions often recur in the same locations as old lesions.

After a period between 10 days and several months, secondary lesions occur, often in a mirror-image configuration on the opposite side of the body. It is very characteristic of this disease that patches which have apparently become dormant may become active again, particularly if treatment is discontinued prematurely.

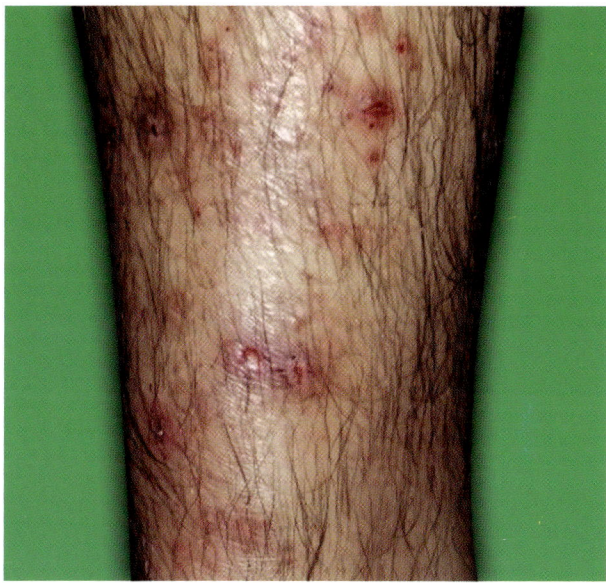

Fig. 11.1: A case of discoid eczema with ovoid crusted lesions on the limb

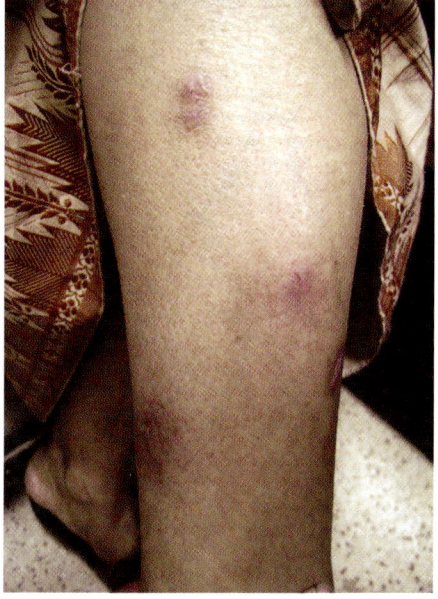

Fig. 11.2: Discoid dry patchs of eczema in a female patient

DIAGNOSIS

A potassium hydroxide wet mount can be obtained to evaluate for dermatophyte infection, but typically no tests are ordered. Skin biopsy findings are non-specific. In the early stages, subacute dermatitis indistinguishable from other forms of eczema with spongiotic vesicles, and a predominant lymphocytic infiltrate. Eosinophils may be observed in the papillary dermis. Chronic lesions demonstrate epidermal hyperplasia, hyperkeratosis, and a pronounced granular cell layer. The papillary dermis may be fibrotic, with a perivenular infiltrate of lymphocytes and monocytes.

DIFFERENTIAL DIAGNOSIS

Diagnostically, this rash can be mistaken for tinea given the annular shape and sharp demarcation with raised peripheral border, but should be differentiated by location, appearance of crusting and scaling surface, lack of central clearing, and past history of eczema. Allergic contact dermatitis, irritant contact dermatitis and aestotic eczema are the other differential diagnoses.

TREATMENT

Treatment is aimed at rehydration of the skin and repair of the epidermal lipid barrier, reduction of inflammation and treatment of any infection stopping the inciting agent (often hot water showers and harsh soaps). Steroids are the most commonly used therapy to reduce inflammation. In the early stages, a potent or very potent steroid may be needed.

Oral, intramuscular, or parenteral steroids may be required in cases of severe, generalized eruptions.

Traditionally, a range of coaltar pastes or ointments were used in the less acute stages, and sometimes a combination of tar and dilute corticosteroid proved useful in long-term management.

Topical immune modulators (tacrolimus and pimecrolimus) also reduce inflammation. These are often initiated a few days after the topical steroid to decrease the risk of a burning sensation that may occur when applied to extremely irritated skin.

When eruptions are generalized and prolonged, phototherapy (generally UV B) may be helpful.

Oral antihistamines or sedatives may help reduce itching and improve sleep.

Oral antibiotics, such as dicloxacillin, cefalexin, or erythromycin, should be used in cases of secondary infection. Swab cultures of the skin guide selection of antibiotics.

Phototherapy may be helpful. Broadband or narrow band UV B is most commonly used, although PUV A (Psoralen + UV A) may be used in severe cases.

An evidence based overview is given in Table 11.1.

Table 11.1: An overview of therapeutic options for discoid eczema

	Topical	Systemic	Phototherapy
First line	Topical corticosteroids ± antibacterial agents (Fucidic acid based preparations)* Emollients Tar-based preparations	Oral antibiotics Oral antihistamines	UVB and PUVA
Second line	Tacrolimus	Cyclosporin Steroids	
Third line		Azathioprine Methotrexate (mycophenolate mofetil)	

*Neomycin based preparations can cause allergic contact dermatitis.

Bibliography

1. Aoyama H, Tanaka M, Hara M, Tabata N, Tagami H. Nummular eczema: An addition of senile xerosis and unique cutaneous reactivities to environmental aeroallergens. Dermatology 1999;199:135–9.

2. Devergie M. Traite Pratique des Maladies de la Peau. 2nd edn [French]. Paris: V. Masson; 1857.

3. Shen Y, Pielop J, Hsu S. Generalized nummular eczema secondary to peginterferon Alfa-2b and ribavirin combination therapy for hepatitis C infection. Arch Dermatol 2005;141:102–3.

4. Wachs GN, Maibach H. Co-operative double blind trial of an antibioticcorticoid combination in impetiginized atopic dermatitis. Br J Dermatol 1976;95:323–8.

12

Pityriasis Alba

DEFINITION

It is derived from word 'pityriasis' means scaly and 'alba' which is a latin word for white although patches are not totally depigmented. This is a pattern of dermatitis in which hypopigmentation is the most conspicuous feature. Although it is common worldwide, its incidence is markedly higher in darker skin phototypes. It is characterized by the presence of ill-defined, scaly, faintly erythematous patches. These lesions eventually subside, leaving hypopigmented areas that then slowly return to normal pigmentation. It is a common skin disorder in children and young adults.

ETIOLOGY

Pityriasis alba (PA) is found almost entirely in preadolescent children. In most instances, the lesions clear at puberty, however persistence into adulthood has been reported (O'Farrell). No known cause of pityriasis alba has been reported. The condition is not contagious, and no infectious agent has been identified.

Leading theories as to the origin of the lesions in pityriasis alba involve atopy and postinflammatory changes, with a large number of patients with pityriasis alba having a history of atopic disease, and atopic patients are being more prone to developing the condition (Martin RF et al, Vinod S et al).

Nutritional deficiency, anemia and parasitic infestations were proposed as contributing factor (Bassaly M et al). In addition, a positive correlation between some personal hygiene habits and PA has been recorded. Long, frequent baths, mechanical exfoliation, and other similar treatments may reduce the level of defensins and skin-protecting factors, contributing to the development of lesions.

CLINICAL FEATURES

It most frequently affects children ages 3 to 16 years. Both sexes are equally susceptible. Pityriasis alba lesions often occur on the face, with the cheek being a particularly common site. In 20% of affected children the neck, arms and shoulders are involved as well as the face. The legs and trunk are less commonly involved. There are three clinical variants of PA: classic (CPA), extensive (EPA), and pigmenting (PPA).The first two variants occur in all skin phototypes. The pigmenting variant is typical of non-Caucasian populations from the Republic of South Africa and the Middle East (Jadotte YT et al).

Classic pityriasis alba: The individual lesion is a rounded, oval or irregular hypopigmented patch which is with indistinct margins. Lesions are often slightly erythematous and have fine scaling (Fig. 12.1). Initially, the erythema may be conspicuous and there may even be minimal serous crusting. Later, the erythema subsides completely, and at the stage at which the lesions are commonly seen by a physician they show only persistent fine scaling and hypopigmentation. It is this that commonly induces the patient to seek advice. The hypopigmentation is most conspicuous in pigmented skin, and in lighter skins may become more evident after sun (Fig. 12.2).

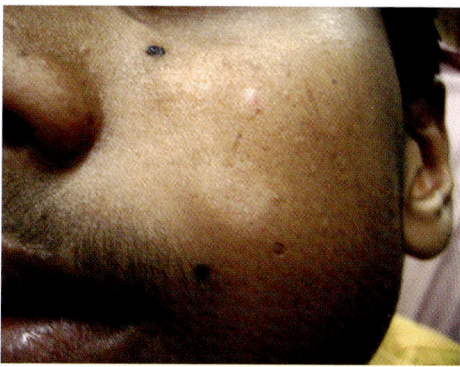

Fig. 12.1: An initial stage of pityriasis alba with fine scaling and an underlying area of hypopigmentation

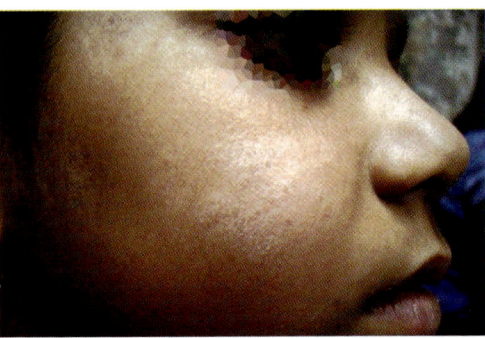

Fig. 12.2: Uniform scaling which eventually heal to leave behind an area of pigmentary loss

Lesions may progress through the following 3 clinical stages:
- Papular (scaling) erythematous
- Papular (scaling) hypochromic
- Smooth hypochromic

Uncommon variants of pityriasis alba are as follows:
- *Pigmenting pityriasis alba:* Typical lesion has a central zone of bluish hyperpigmentation surrounded by a hypopigmented, slightly scaly halo of variable width; the lesions are usually confined to the face and are often associated with dermatophyte infection. The pigmented area is attributed to melanin deposits in dermis. One-third of the patients have concurrent classic pityriasis alba.
- *Extensive pityriasis alba:* It is more commonly seen in adults. Differentiated from the classic form by the generalized involvement often involoving the inferior torso in symmetric fashion, the absence of a preceding inflammatory phase, and histologically, the absence of spongiosis.

Debate exists as to the validity of the term extensive pityriasis alba, which some believe to be a confusing misnomer applied to a pathoetiologically different entity. Some authors believe that extensive pityriasis alba overlaps with another condition, described as "progressive and extensive hypomelanosis" in persons of mixed racial background and also reported as "progressive and confluent hypomelanosis of the melanodermic metis" or "creole dyschromia." The alternate name of "progressive extensive hypomelanosis" has been proposed (Di Lernia V).

Diagnosis

The age incidence, the fine scaling and the distribution of the lesions usually suggest the diagnosis. A workup, as follows, may be undertaken to exclude other causes of hypopigmentation:

- *Wood's light examination:* May help in determining the presence of vitiligo, which will glow more brightly and have edges with sharper demarcation.

- *Skin biopsy:* The histological changes are acanthosis and mild spongiosis, with moderate hyperkeratosis and patchy parakeratosis. There may be follicular plugging, spongiosis and sebaceous gland atrophy, and irregular pigmentation by melanin of the basal layer of epidermis. Irregular pigmentation in the late stage has been recorded in all patients and is thus considered to be characteristic of PA.

DIFFERENTIAL DIAGNOSIS

- Post-inflammatory hypopigmentation
- Nevus anemicus
- Nevus depigmentosus
- Tuberous sclerosis
- Vitiligo
- Tinea versicolor
- Mycosis fungoides

MANAGEMENT

Pityriasis alba is generally self-limited, and the prognosis is good, with eventual complete repigmentation. No long-term residual effects are expected. Treatment consists primarily of good general skin care and education of a young patient's parents about the benign nature of this self-limited disorder. Supportive measures such as decrease sun exposure, use of sunscreens and reduction of frequency and temperature of baths should be recommended. Therapy may also include the following:

- *Low-potency topical steroids (e.g. hydrocortisone):* May help in stage 1 and stage 2 of pityriasia alba and may accelerate repigmentation of existing lesions. However, their use should be limited to avoid long-term skin atrophy and steroid changes.

- *Emollient cream:* Used to reduce the scaling of lesions, especially on the face.

- *Psoralen plus ultraviolet light A (PUVA) photochemotherapy:* May be used to help with repigmentation in extensive cases; recurrence rate is high after treatment is stopped.

- *Tacrolimus ointment 0.1% and pimecrolimus cream 1%:* Have been reported to be beneficial in the treatment of pityriasis alba (Rigopoulos D et al, Fujita WH et al). It is effective when applied to hypopigmented areas in the third stage of disease as it has an activating effect on tyrosinase and enhancement of melanin biosynthesis.

- *Laser therapy:* Treatment with a 308-nm excimer laser twice a week has been shown to be effective against pityriasis alba (Al-Mutairi N et al).

Bibliography

1. Al-Mutairi N, Hadad AA. Efficacy of 308 nm xenon chloride excimer laser in pityriasis alba. *Dermatol Surg* 2012 Apr. 38(4):604–9.

2. Bassaly M, Miale A. Studies on pityriasis alba—a common facial skin lesion in Egyptian children. *Arch Dermatol* 1963;88: 88–91.

3. Di Lernia V, Ricci C. On atopic and idiopatic extensive pityriasis alba. Pediatr Dermatol. 2007 Sep-Oct. 24(5):578–9.

4. Fujita WH, McCormick CL, Parneix-Spake A. An exploratory study to evaluate the efficacy of pimecrolimus cream 1% for the treatment of pityriasis alba. *Int J Dermatol* 2007 Jul 46(7):700–5.

5. Jadotte YT, Janniger CK. Pityriasis alba revisited: perspectives on an enigmatic disorder of childhood. *Cutis* 2011;87:66–72.

6. Martin RF, Lugo-Somolinos A, Sanchez JL. Clinicopathologic study on pityriasis alba. *Bol Asoc Med P R* 1990 Oct. 82(10):463–5.

7. O'Farrell NM. Pityriasis alba. *Arch Dermatol* 1956;73: 376–377.

8. Rigopoulos D, Gregoriou S, Charissi C, Kontochristopoulos G, Kalogeromitros D, Georgala S. Tacrolimus ointment 0.1% in pityriasis alba: an open-label, randomized, placebo-controlled study. *Br J Dermatol*. 2006 Jul. 155(1):152–5.

9. Vinod S, Singh G, Dash K, Grover S. Clinico epidemiological study of pityriasis alba. *Indian J Dermatol Venereol Leprol*. 2002 Nov-Dec. 68(6):338–40.

13

Hand Eczema

Hands are an important part of our body as they help us in our daily activities and also have aesthetic importance. They can become a cause of serious disability when afflicted with chronic disease and can lead to significant psychosocial impairment.

"Hand dermatitis/eczema" is predominant involvement of the hands with eczema. It is different from widespread eczema with simultaneous hand involvement.

ETIOLOGY

Hand eczema has multifactorial etiology (Table 13.1). Both exogenous (extrinsic) and endogenous (intrinsic) factors may be involved in the pathogenesis of hand eczema. There are a few predictive factors for hand eczema of which a history of childhood eczema was the most important predictive factor for hand eczema. Other factors are listed in Box 13.1.

Table 13.1: The etiologic classification of hand eczema

Classification of hand eczema
1 Irritant contact dermatitis
2 Allergic contact dermatitis
3 Atopic hand dermatitis
4 Protein contact dermatitis
5 Hybrid hand eczema
6 Unclassified

Box 1: Predictive factors for hand eczema

- History of childhood eczema
- Female gender
- Occupational exposure
- History of asthma and/or hay fever
- Service occupation (e.g. professional cleaners)

Meding B, Swanbeck G: Contact Dermatitis 23:154, 1990.

Irritant Contact Dermatitis (ICD)

In ICD, eczema occurs without prior sensitization. Exposure to irritants impairs the barrier functions of the skin. ICD of the hands is frequently seen in female cleaners, hospital workers, hairdressers, painters and laborers. Most of the patients have a history of exposure to "wet" work. Common irritants are detergents, solvents, alkalies, abrasives. ICD can be acute (single external exposure to irritant for short duration) or chronic (repeated exposure to irritants over a prolonged period) (Fig. 13.1a).

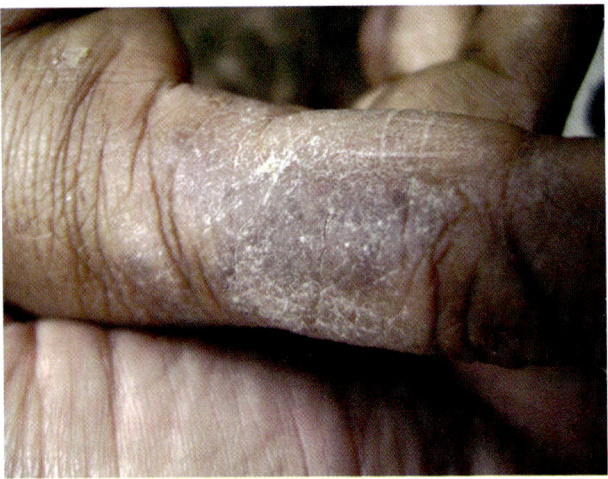

Fig. 13.1a: A chronic patch of eczema on the finger

Allergic Contact Dermatitis

It is a delayed type hypersensitivity reaction an allergen or chemical in which prior sensitization occurs. Allertic contact dermatitis (ACD) occurs 1 to 2 days after contact and is initially localized to the site of exposure. Vegetables, detergents, soaps, topical drugs, metals, industrial agents, nuts are the major allergens found in Indian series. The chemicals responsible are nickel (tools, jewellery), chromate (leather, cement), rubber additives (in gloves), preservatives (in creams). Figure 13.1b depicts a patient with allergic contact dermatitis to gloves. Oral ingestion of allergen (e.g nickel) can also provoke hand eczema, though rare (Jensen et al). A list of common allergens implicated is given in Box 13.2.

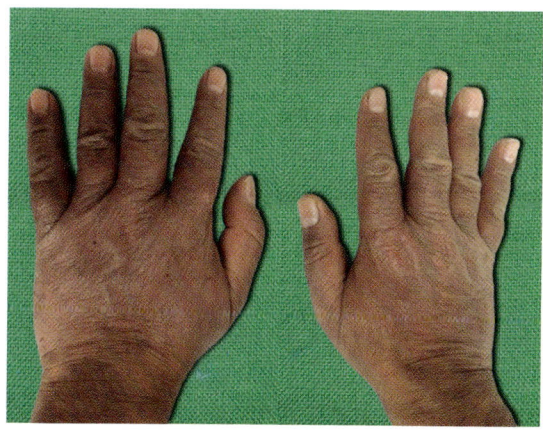

Fig. 13.1b: Allergic dermatitis to gloves in a health care worker with marked involvement of the dorsum of the hands

Box 13.2: A list of common allergens and the common objects implicated	
Nickel	Door knobs, handles on kitchen utensils, scissors, knitting needles, industrial equipment, hairdressing equipment, metallic mobile phones
Potassium dichromate	Cement, leather articles (gloves), industrial machines, oils
Rubber	Gloves, industrial equipment (hoses, belts, cables)
Fragrances	Cosmetics, soaps, lubricants, topical medications
Formaldehyde	Wash and wear fabrics, paper, cosmetics, embalming fluid
Lanolin	Topical lubricants and medications, cosmetics.

Atopic Hand Eczema

Patients often have a history of asthma, hay fever or childhood eczema. The following factors predict the occurrence of hand eczema in adults with a history of atopic dermatitis:

- Hand dermatitis before age 15
- Persistent eczema on the body
- Dry or itchy skin in adult life
- Widespread atopic dermatitis in childhood

Many people with atopic dermatitis develop hand eczema independently of exposure to irritants, but such exposure causes additional irritant contact dermatitis. Hands are the most frequent site to be involved in adults with atopic dermatitis. The clinical features that point to an atopic etiology are involvement of dorsal hand surfaces and the volar wrist (Simpson et al). Out of all types of hand eczema, atopic hand eczema has the worst prognosis (Meding at al).

Protein Contact Eczema

It is a type I hypersensitivity reaction mediated by Ig E (allergen specific) in a sensitised individual. It is clinically characterised by chronic or recurrent dermatitis usually of the fingertips. Urticarial or vesicular lesions occur within minutes of contact with incriminated proteins (e.g fruits, vegetables, spices, grains). Repeated exposure causes eczema. It is usually seen in cooks, caterers, food handlers, housewives).

Hybrid Hand Eczema

It combines aspects of ICD, ACD and atopic dermatitis.

Unclassified

In patients with chronic hand eczema, it is difficult to characterise the cause.

Hand eczema can also be classified based on the morphology of lesions (Table 13.2) and the stage of the disease (Table 13.3). Though the morphology is commonly relied upon, they can have multiple etiologies and thus it is important for the clinician to elicit the causes in each type.

Table 13.2: Morphological classification of hand eczema

Morphological classification of hand eczema

1. Recurrent vesicular/dyshidrotic hand eczema or pompholyx
2. Hyperkeratotic/tylotic hand eczema
3. Nummular hand eczema
4. Wear and tear/asteatotic/housewives' dermatitis/dermatitis palmaris sicca.
5. Chronic fingertip eczema/pulpitis
6. Ring eczema
7. Recurrent focal palmer peeling
8. Apron eczema
9. Chronic acral dermatitis
10. Interdigital (webspace) eczema
11. Gut/Slaughterhouse eczema
12. Patchy/papulosquamous eczema

Table 13.3: Classification of hand eczema based on the stage of disease

Classification of hand eczema based on the stage of disease	*Clinical features*
1. Acute	Erythema, edema, vesiculation, exudation, bullae formation
2. Subacute	Erythema, papules and crusting
3. Chronic	Lichenification (thickening of skin, accentuated skin markings, hyperpigmentation)

Pompholyx/Recurrent Vesicular Dyshidrotic Hand Eczema*

In this variant of hand eczema, deep-seated "sago-like" clear vesicles appear on palms and sides of fingers (cheiropompholyx). Lesions can also occur on plantar aspect of feet (podopompholyx). There is no associated erythema. Pompholyx accounts for 5–20% of all cases of hand eczema (Fig. 13.2). The condition is extremely itchy. A prickling sensation precedes the attacks. Resolution occurs in 2–3 weeks with dequamation. Summer exacerbation may be seen. Pompholyx has multifactorial etiology most important of which is atopy. Other factors are sweat gland dysfunction, exposure to irritants (soluble oils), allergens (nickel, chromium,

---

*Also see Chapter 15.

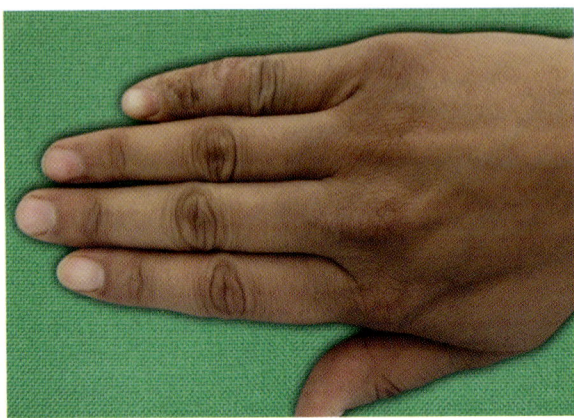

Fig. 13.2: The fifth digit depicts an area of pompholyx in the healing stage

cobalt, dichromates, perfumes, fragrances). Oral contraceptive pills (OCP), aspirin intake and smoking increase the risk of pompholyx. Differential diagnosis includes pustular psoriasis and erythema multiforme.

Hyperkeratotic (Tylotic) Hand Eczema*

It is characterised by well-defined hyperkeratotic plaques on the palms and palmar surfaces of the fingers. Simultaneous involvement of plantar aspect of feet may be seen. It is common in middle aged men. An Indian study (Minocha et al) has revealed contact sensitivity (to vegetables, detergents, metals, rubber) in patch test done in patients with hyperkeratotic hand eczema (Minocha et al). The condition is resistant to treatment. Figure 13.3 shows a patient with hyperkeratotic hand eczema. Psoriasis is a close differential diagnosis. However, the latter has well demarcated lesions that are non-itchy.

Wear and Tear/Asteatotic/Housewives' Dermatitis

Various factors are involved in its pathogenesis. These are exposure to irritants, asteatosis, trauma or friction. It is seen in occupations that involve wet work and exposure to detergents. Hence common in housewives and cleaners. The palmar skin of bilateral hands becomes dry, cracked and criss-crossed. Exudation and pruritus are not seen.

---

*Also see Chapter 14.

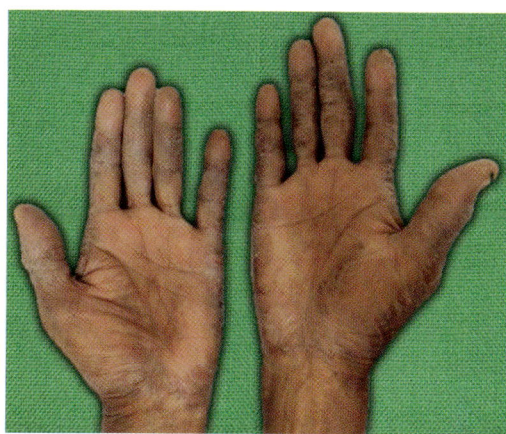

Fig. 13.3: Symmetrical chronic eczematous patchs on the palms of a patient with tylotic eczema

Discoid Eczema

It is characterised by round to oval plaques of eczema that have a well demarcated edge. Various factors involved in its pathogenesis are atopy, infection, trauma, allergic sensitivity and emotional stress. Discoid eczema of the hands generally affects the dorsal aspect of hands or the back or sides of fingers (Fig. 13.4). Single plaque is seen initially followed by appearance of secondary

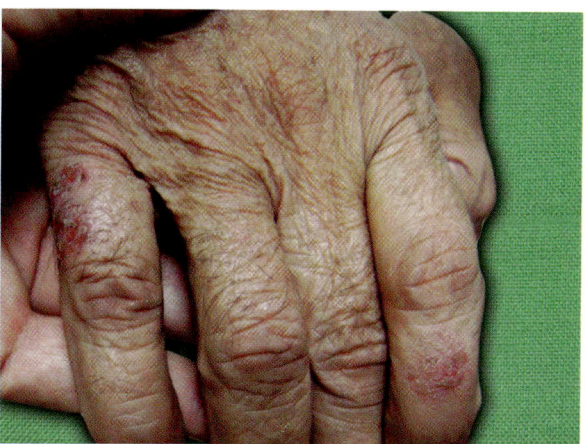

Fig. 13.4: Oval patchs of discoid eczema on the dorsal aspect of the hand

lesions on fingers or forearms. Secondary infection with *S. aureus* may occur.

Fingertip Eczema/Pulpitis

Eczema develops on the palmar surface of the tips of fingers. Skin becomes dry, cracked and fissures can develop (Fig. 13.5). The condition can be due to irritant or allergic contact dermatitis.

Ring Eczema

A patch of eczema develops under a ring and can spread to the adjacent skin. It occurs due to accumulation of soaps and detergents under the ring.

Apron Eczema

It involves the proximal palmar aspect of two adjacent fingers. It can extend onto the palmar skin over the metacarpophalangeal joints. It is usually seen in women. It can be due to irritant or allergic contact dermatitis.

Chronic Acral Dermatitis

It is characterised by hyperkeratotic papulovesicular eczema of hands and feet. It is usually seen in middle aged patients. The condition is associated with elevated IgE levels.

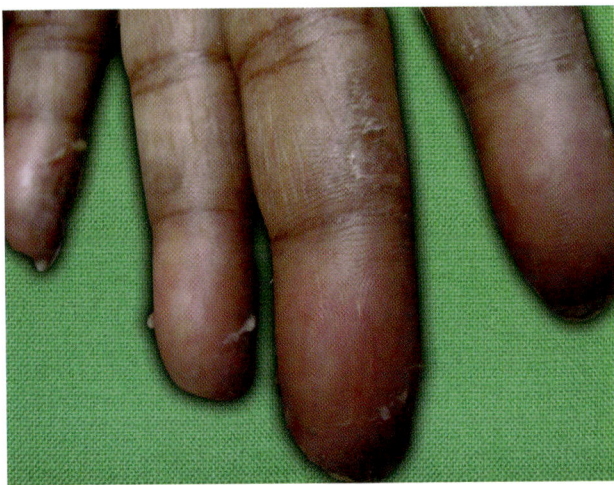

Fig. 13.5: Fissuring with desquamation in a case of fingertip eczema

Gut/Slaughterhouse Eczema

It is seen in people who deal with animal carcasses in slaughterhouses. Vesicular plaque starts from the webs of fingers and then spreads to the sides. The condition is usually transient.

Recurrent Focal Palmar Peeling

Keratolysis exfoliativa or recurrent focal palmar peeling is a common, chronic, asymptomatic, noninflammatory bilateral peeling of the palms of the hands (Fig. 13.6) and occasionally soles of the feet; its cause is unknown. The eruption is most common during the summer months and is often associated with sweaty palms and soles. Scaling starts simultaneously from several points on the palms or soles with 2 or 3 mm of round scales that appear to have originated from a ruptured vesicle. Some believe it to be associated with dyshidrosis and is believed to be a mild cases of pompholyx.

DIFFERENTIAL DIAGNOSIS

Hand eczema may be confused with other dermatological conditions (Table 13.4).

Assessment of Severity

Various scoring indices have been developed to assess the severity of hand eczema but are hardly used in clinical practice. The hand

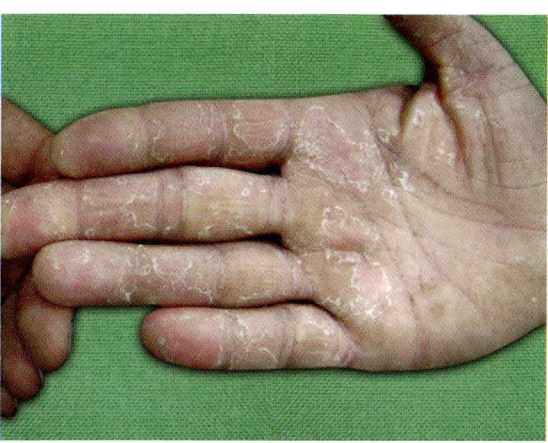

Fig. 13.6: Focal and annular patch of scaling on the palms in a case of keratolysis exfoliativa

Table 13.4: Differential diagnosis of hand eczema

Location	Redness and scaling	Vesicles	Pustules
Dorsum of hand	Atopic dermatitis Irritant contact dermatitis Lichen simplex chronicus Nummular eczema Psoriasis Tinea	Id reaction Scabies (web spaces)	Bacterial infection Psoriasis Scabies (web spaces) Tinea
Palmar surface	Fingertip eczema Hyperkeratotic eczema Recurrent focal palmar peeling Psoriasis Tinea	Allergic contact dermatitis Pompholyx (dyshidrosis)	Bacterial infection Pompholyx (dyshidrosis) Psoriasis

eczema severity index (HECSI) was developed as a clinical grading tool but is mainly used for research.

DIAGNOSIS

One should elicit history pertaining to mode of onset, frequency and duration of symptoms and any seasonal exacerbation. Details about exposure at workplace, history of contact with chemicals, oils, wet work should be sought. Exposure to allergens during household work as well as during leisure activities should be inquired. Atopy should be ruled out on history. Patient should be asked about treatment taken and any exposure to medication.

The type of lesions and their distribution should be noted on cutaneous examination. Involvement of other body parts should be checked. A few patients, where diagnosis is doubtful might require few investigations as elicited in Table 13.5.

PREVENTION

1. *Appropriate changes in lifestyle* should be carried out to minimise exposure to irritants and allergens. Patients in high risk occupations like cleaners, hairdressers, healthcare workers, food

Table 13.5: Provides the diagnostic work-up for a patient with hand eczema

Investigation	
1. KOH mount	Done from active border of the lesion to rule out tinea.
2. Gram stain	To rule out secondary bacterial infections in cases with oozing and purulent discharge.
3. Absolute eosinophil count (AEC) and serum immunoglo-bulins	To rule out atopic diathesis
4. Skin biopsy	In doubtful cases to differentiate form conditions like psoriasis.
5. Patch testing	In cases of suspected ACD or cases failing to respond to treatment, chronic hand and foot eczema.
6. 24 hour patch testing	With detergent and soap solutions (8% v/v) for patient in whom detergents are a cause of hand eczema (e.g. housewives, cleaners).
7. Prick test	In cases of suspected protein contact dermatitis or contact urticaria caused by latex or fish proteins.
8. RAST	Radioallergosorbent test.

handlers should be identified and educated appropriately. Patients should be informed about high risk factors like wet work and low humidity.

2. *Various protective measures* can be adopted at the workplace and at home. Barrier creams can be used before and during work. These contain aluminium chlorhydrate, zinc oxide, talcum and have to be applied on intact skin. They decrease penetration of irritants. Alcohol-based hand rubs (containing emollients) and mild skin cleansers can be used for cleaning hands after work (instead of soaps and detergents). Gloves can be used to avoid exposure to irritants and allergens.

3. *Emollients and moisturizers* should be used liberally after work. They moisturise the skin and prevent drying. They provide

protection form irritants and help restore the skin barrier. However, urea containing moisturisers should be avoided as they increase skin permeability and might enhance penetration of few irritants (Wohlrab et al). Emollients and moisturisers are the mainstay of prevention and treatment of chronic hand eczema.

TREATMENT (see Table 13.6)

Table 13.6: A summary of the treatment options in hand eczema

Topical	Systemic	Others
Moisturizers	Corticosteroids	Phototherapy
Keratolytics	Retinoids	Radiotherapy
Steroids	Immunosuppressants	
Calcineurin inhibitors		
Retinoids		
Coal tar		
Botulinum toxin		

Topical Therapy

1. *Moisturizers:* They help to restore the skin barrier that is affected by eczema. They should be applied frequently and liberally. Ointments may be preferred over creams. The latter contain preservatives that can be sensitising and emulsifiers that can act as irritants. White petrolatum is the moisturiser of choice as it is both an emollient and a barrier cream.

2. *Keratolytics:* These can be used in cases of chronic hand eczema especially the hyperkeratotoic type. Keratolytics include salicylic acid (up to 20%) and urea (5–10%). Urea increases the water binding capacity of skin. However, it might enhance the penetration of few chemicals as mentioned previously.

3. *Topical steroids:* Topical steroids and moisturizers are the mainstay of treatment of hand eczema. Potent topical steroids can be used initially for one month followed by maintenance therapy three times per week (Drake et al). Potent steroids are more effective than moderately potent steroids (Moller et al). They also reduce the risk of recurrences. However, long term use can cause side effects like skin atrophy (causing further

weakening of skin barrier), tachyphylaxis and adrenal suppression. Calcineurin inhibitors can be added along with a moderately-potent topical steroid to reduce the side effects. Worsening of eczema suggests contact allergy to steroid cream or other ingredients and patch test should be done in such cases.

4. *Topical calcineurin inhibitors (tacrolimus/pimecrolimus):* These are immunomodulators and act as steroid sparing agents. These are not licenced for the treatment of hand eczema, however trials have shown favorable results. These can also be combined with moderate potent steroids for maintenance therapy. Side effects include mild burning sensation that is transient and sensitivity to light.

5. *Topical retinoids:* Topical Bexarotene gel has shown good efficacy in a randomised trial in patients with chronic severe hand eczema (Hanifin et al). It can cause side effects like irritation of skin, burning sensation and flare of dermatitis.

6. *Topical coal tar:* It can be used in patients with subacute and chronic eczema. It has anti-inflammatory, anti-proliferative and antipruritic effects.

7. *Botulinum toxin:* It can be used as an adjunctive therapy for vesicular eczema associated with hyperhidrosis.

Others

1. **Phototherapy:** It is widely used for hand eczema. PUV B, broad band UV B, UV A1 all are used in the treatment. A study has shown that PUV A is more efficacious than UV B in chronic eczema of hands. However, a few side effects, e.g. nausea (due to oral methoxsalen), edema and pain can occur. Long-term side effects include increased risk of skin cancer.

2. **Radiotherapy:** Grenz rays and superficial X-rays both have been used in the treatment of hand eczema. Superficial X-rays penetrate deeper and hence are more effective. But Grenz rays are safer.

Systemic Therapy

1. *Oral corticosteroids:* These can be used for the management of acute flares. However, side effects preclude use of oral steroids for long-term.

2. *Oral retinoids:* There is a little evidence supporting the use of oral retinoids in hand eczema. One study reported 50% improvement

with oral acitretin 40 mg daily in patients with hyperkeratotic hand eczema (Pederson et al). Hence, combined therapy may be used.

Alitretinoin (9-*cis*-retinoic acid) is an endogenous physical retinoid that is structurally similar to isotretinoin. It is the only evidence-based treatment option for patients with severe chronic hand eczema who are unresponsive to topical steroids. Randomized controlled trials (RCTs) have shown good response with alitretinoin 10–30 mg once daily for up to 24 weeks (Ruzicka et al). Also side effects are less compared to other retinoids. Common side effects with alitretinoin are headache, mucosal and cutaneous dryness, reduction in TSH levels and hypertriglyceridemia. When using alitretinoin, it is important to counsel the female patients regarding contraception during treatment and one month after stopping treatment.

3. *Immunosuppressants:* These are used only in patients who have severe chronic hand eczema unresponsive to other treatments.

Cyclosporine is the most frequently used especially in patients with history of atopic eczema. It is given in a dose of 2.5–3 mg/kg/day and gradually tapered over a few months. Serum electrolytes, creatinine and blood pressure should be monitored during treatment.

Azathioprine is used in a dose of 2 mg/kg/day. Patients with atopic dermatitis respond well to azathioprine.

Methotrexate, in a dose of 5–20 mg once weekly, has been found to be effective in hand eczema (Shaffrali et al). It should be remembered that all immunosuppressive agents pose a risk of serious side effects (hematological toxicity, hepatic dysfunction, opportunistic infections, etc.) and should only be used in unresponsive patients.

Bibliography

1. Drake LA, Dinehart SM, Farmer ER, et al. Guidelines of care for the use of topical glicocorticosteroids. J Am Acad Dermatol 1996; 35:615–9.

2. Hanifin JM, Stevens V, Sheth P, et al. Novel treatment of chronic severe hand dermatitis with bexarotene gel. Br J Dermatol 2004; 150(3):545–53.

3. Jensen CS, Menne T, Johansen JD. Systemic contact dermatitis after oral exposure to nickel: a review with a modified meta-analysis. Contact Dermatitis 2006; 54:79–86.

4. Meding B, Swanbeck G. Epidemiology of different types of hand eczema in an industrial city. Acta Derm Venereol 1989; 69: 227–33.

5. Meding B, Swanbeck G: Contact Dermatitis 23:154, 1990.

6. Minocha YC, Dogra A, Sood VK. Contact sensitivity in palmer hyperkeratotic dermatitis. Indian J Dermatol Venerol Leprol 1983;59: 60–3.

7. Moller H, Svartholm H, Dahl G. Intermittent maintenance therapy in chronic hand eczema with clobetasol propionate and fluprednilen acetate. Curr Med Res Opin 1983;8:640–4.

8. Ruzicka T, Lynde CW, Jemec GB, Diepgen T, Berth-Jones J, Coenraads PJ, et al. Efficacy and safety of oral alitretinoin (9-*cis* retinoic acid) in patients with severe chronic hand eczema refractory to topical corticosteroids: Results of a randomized, double-blind, placebo-controlled, multicentre trial. Br J Dermatol 2008;158:808–17.

9. Shaffrali FC, Colver GB, Messenger AG, Gawkrodger DJ. Experience with low-dose methotrexate for the treatment of eczema in the elderly. J Am Acad Dermatol 2003;48:417–9.

10. Simpson EL, Thompson MM, Hanifin JM. Prevalence and morphology of hand eczema in patients with atopic dermatitis. Dermatitis 2006; 17:123–27.

11. Thestrup-Pederson K, Andersen KE, Menne T, Veien NK. Treatment of hyperkeratotic dermatitis of the palms (eczema keratoticum) with oral acitretin. A single-blind placebo-controlled study. Acta Derm Venereol 2001;81:353–5.

12. Wohlrab W. The influence of urea on the penetration kinetics of topically applied corticosteroids Acta Derm Venereol (Stockh) 1984;64:233–8.

14

Hyperkeratotic Eczema of the Palms

Hyperkeratotic eczema of the palms (also called hyperkeratotic hand eczema) is a relatively frustrating recalcitrant form of hand dermatitis which more often than not gets labeled as psoriasis and has then different connotations for the clinician and the patient.

CLINICAL FEATURES

Although the nomenclature and the clinical and pathological presentations of the variants of hand eczema often overlap and render the diagnostic classification imprecise, this condition presents as chronic, scaly, slightly erythematous, hyperkeratotic, fissure-prone plaques on the palms (Fig. 14.1a). Typically, plaques are discrete, with relatively sharp margins (Fig. 14.1b). They have a multifocal and symmetrical distribution. Sometimes the plaques coalesce together to cover most of the palmar surface. They typically occur on the central palms (Fig. 14.1a). The border of the palms and the volar surfaces of the fingers may also be involved (Fig. 14.2). The eruption tends to spare dorsal hand and fingertips. Plantar involvement is seen in some cases. The eruption may be asymptomatic but in nearly half of the patients, it is itchy. When fissures are present, it may be painful.

ETIOLOGY

Hyperkeratotic eczema of the palms is considered an endogenous dermatitis. The etiology is unknown, the patients usually have no relevant irritant exposure or contact sensitization, patch tests are usually negative, and the incidence of atopy is not greater than in the general population. The prevalence of psoriasis in close

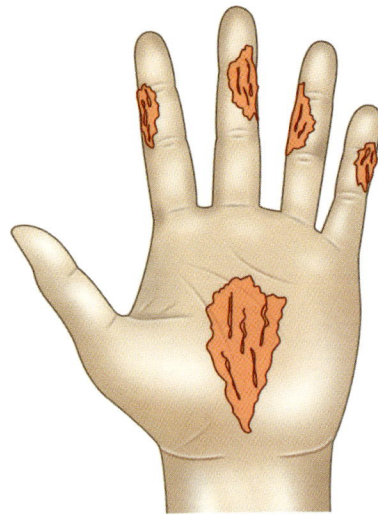

Fig. 14.1a: A depiction of the sites of involvement in hyperkeratotic eczema including the palms and volar aspects of fingers

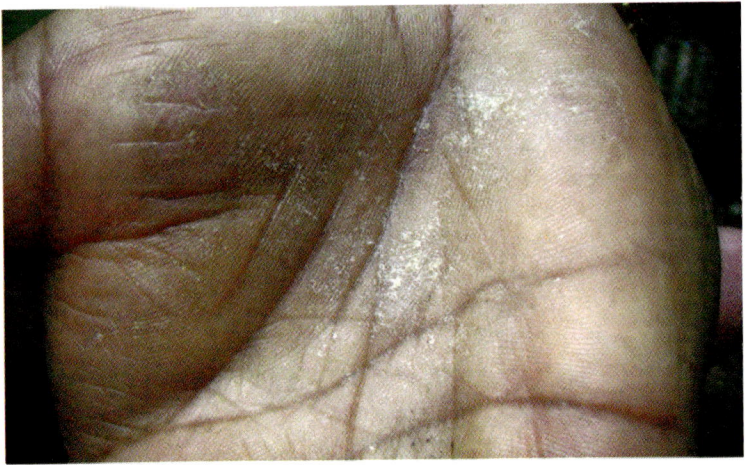

Fig. 14.1b: A hyperkeratotic plaque in the center of the palm

relatives does not differ from what can be found in the general population.

There is a debate about whether this is merely a variant of psoriasis as the histologic features of palmoplantar psoriasis and eczema overlap with each other.

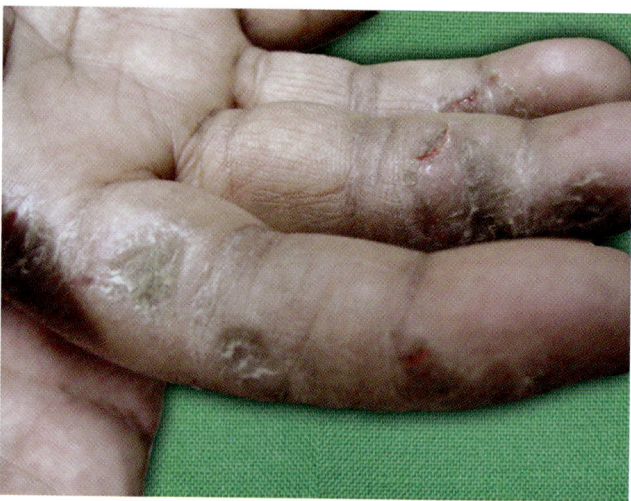

Fig. 14.2: Fissured, thick plaques on the fingers

TREATMENT

Although hyperkeratotic (HK) hand dermatitis is not considered a form of contact dermatitis, traditionally, the recommendation is to avoid irritants and to encourage aggressive use of emollients. Many patients suffer disease exacerbations from excessive exposure to hot water and harsh detergents. Use of cool water, mild soaps, adequate protection, and an emollient hand cream is critical to prevent relapses in these patients.

Topical Agents

a. Topical corticosteroids are usually first-line treatment for hyperkeratotic hand dermatitis

b. Topical vitamin D_3 derivatives have been used with some success in treatment of hyperkeratotic hand eczema.

c. Other topical treatments such as tar, calcineurin inhibitors (tacrolimus and pimecrolimus), and retinoids (bexarotene and tazarotene) have been used successfully in treating chronic hand eczema

d. In patients with significant hyperkeratosis, topical lactic acid 5–12% or urea 10–40% preparations may be added to the above treatment. These will reduce the scale and enhance the penetration of the active agents.

Phototherapy

Various forms of phototherapy have been used though PUV A is a better option and safer if used topically in the so called "paint PUV A" protocol. Though there are reports of the use of Nb UV B, its penetration is less than UV A and is thus would not be as effective as PUV A, though some trials report an equipotent effect.

Systemic Agents

Acitretin is considered an effective treatment for hyperkeratotic hand eczema and is especially useful for thinning out thick hyperkeratotic areas and making the lesions more susceptible to other treatments such as topical agents and phototherapy. A dose of 30 mg daily is good enough for a predictable response.

In severe refractory cases, *cyclosporine* A 3–5 mg/kg, *mycophenolate* mofetil 2 gm/day, or methotrexate 10–25 mg once weekly, may be considered. Alitretinoin (not available in India) may also be a highly effective therapeutic for refractory disease of the hyperkeratotic presentation of hand dermatitis.

Bibliography

1. Chopra A, Maninder, Gill SS. Hyperkeratosis of palms and soles: clinical study. Indian J Dermatol Venereol Leprol. 1997;63(2):85–8.

2. Diepgen TL, Andersen KE, Brandao FM, Bruze M, Bruynzeel DP, Frosch P, et al. Hand eczema classification: a cross-sectional, multicentre study of the aetiology and morphology of hand eczema. Br J Dermatol. 2009;160(2):353–8.

3. Hersle K, Mobacken H. Hyperkeratotic dermatitis of the palms. Br J Dermatol. 1982;107(2):195–201.

4. Pettey AA, Balkrishnan R, Rapp SR, Fleischer AB, Feldman SR. Patients with palmoplantar psoriasis have more physical disability and discomfort than patients with other forms of psoriasis: implications for clinical practice. J Am Acad Dermatol. 2003;49(2): 271–5.

5. Steven R. Feldman and Arash Taheri. Hyperkeratotic eczema of the palms. A. Alikhan et al. (eds.), Textbook of Hand Eczema, © Springer: Verlag Berlin Heidelberg 2014.

6. Veien NK, Hattel T, Laurberg G. Hand eczema: causes, course, and prognosis I. Contact Dermatitis. 2008;58(6):330–4.

15

Acute and Recurrent Vesicular Hand Eczema (Syn Pompholyx)

Acute and recurrent vesicular hand eczema is defined as the infrequent or repeated eruption of vesicles on the palms, palmar aspects of the fingers, and/or sides of the fingers (Fig. 15.1a) that cannot be explained by contact with external contactants.

Acute and vesicular hand dermatitis should be preferred over pompholyx and dyshidrosis as we still do not know what causes this intriguing clinical manifestation.

CLINICAL TYPES

The term acute and recurrent vesicular hand eczema has been chosen, because there appear to be two clinical types of this dermatitis. One type is explosive, with eruptions of severe vesiculation (Fig. 15.1b) or even bullous lesions. This type is rare and is representative of the initial descriptions of the dermatosis made in the late nineteenth century. Most of the cases described over the past 30 years are of a less severe type, with repeated eruptions of tiny, severely pruritic vesicles (Figs 15.1c and d).

ETIOLOGY

A variety of causes have been described with varying levels of evidence and they constitute a useful list to run through before hurriedly labeling the patient as an idiopathic disorder (Table 15.1). A study by Guillet MH found that the common causes were mycosis (10.0%); allergic contact pompholyx (67.5%), with cosmetic and hygiene products as the main factor (31.7%), followed by metals (16.7%); and internal reactivation from drug, food, or haptenic (nickel) origin (6.7%). The remaining 15.0% of patients were classified as idiopathic patients, but all were atopic.

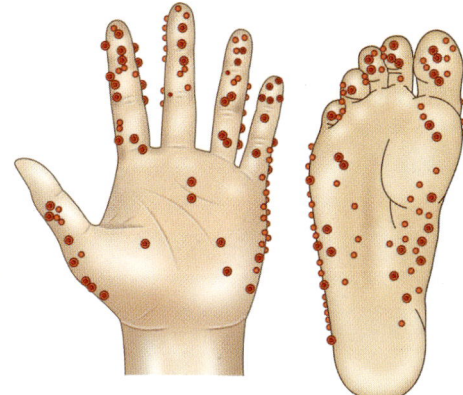

Fig. 15.1a: Pompholyx. A depiction of multiple "sago grain" like vesicles on the sides of fingers

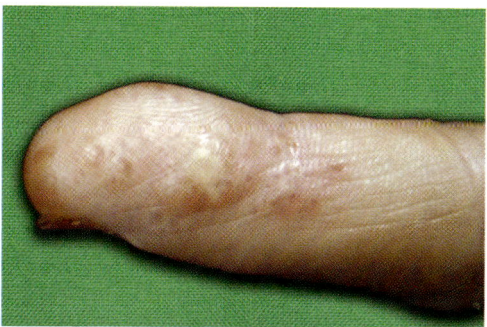

Fig. 15.1b: Large vesicles coalescing into a bulla in a case of vesicular hand eczema

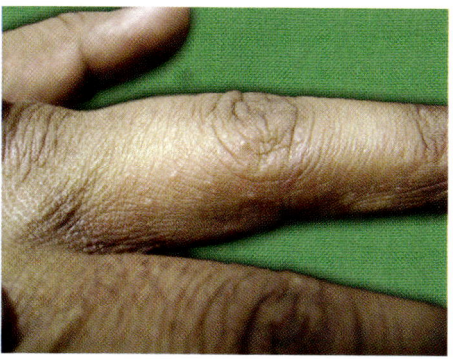

Fig. 15.1c: Vesicular eruption on the fingers

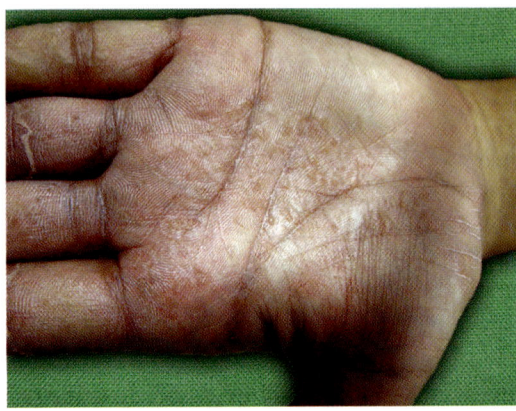

Fig. 15.1d: A patient with a history of recurrent vesicles on the palmar aspect

TREATMENT

The most important aspect of the management of acute and recurrent vesicular hand eczema is the determination of the cause of the eruptions where the list below (Table 15.1) can be a useful initial exercise.

The history should include information about external and possible systemic exposures. Vesicular eruptions have been described as occurring less than 1 h after exposure to proteins in

Table 15.1: Possible causes of acute and recurrent vesicular hand eczema

Atopy

Dermatophytid

Drug reactions

Systemic contact dermatitis

Allergic contact dermatitis
(*garlic, compositae plants, balsam of Peru*)

Metals
(*Dental metals, orthodontic treatment, Ni, chromium*)

Ingested metals
(*Ni, chromium*)

Food
(*Tuna, coffee, tomato, pineapple, American cheese, milk, egg, wheat, lamb, chocolate, and chicken.*)

persons with protein contact dermatitis. Oral challenge with nickel has caused vesicular palmar eruptions after 1–3 days in nickel-sensitive patients. A history of exposures up to **3 days** before the eruption of vesicular hand eczema is, therefore, an essential element in the diagnosis of this condition. The history should include information regarding dermatophytosis of the feet, particularly that caused by *T. mentagrophytes*. Patients with recurrent vesicular hand eczema should ideally be patch tested with a standard tray, including the metals nickel, cobalt, and chromium, as well as balsam of Peru and perfume ingredients. When protein contact dermatitis is suspected, prick testing and prick-prick testing should be carried out with suspected food items.

If a diet trials is initiated it should last from **1 to 3 months**. If improvement is not apparent, the diet trial should be discontinued. If improvement is seen, the diet should be moderated to make life easier for the patient.

A list of agents useful in the treatment is given in Box 15.1, though in most cases a relapsing course is seen, a suggested line of management is given in Table 15.2.

Treatments	*Evidence level*[b]
Botulinum toxin A	3[c]
Immunosuppressants (azathioprine, methotrexate, cyclosporine (ciclosporin), mycophenolate mofetil, corticosteroids, etc.	4a[c]
Retinoids (alitretinoin)	2
PUVA	2
Radiotherapy	4a
Selective UVB phototherapy	3
Tap water iontophoresis	3[c]
Topical corticosteroids	2
Topical calcineurin inhibitors	2
Topical bexarotene plus mid-potency corticosteroid	2
UVA-I	2

PUVA psoralen plus UVA

Level 1: evidence is available for meta-analysis from several randomized controlled studies; level 2: evidence is available from at least one randomized controlled trial; level 4; evidence is available from good methodologic studies without randomization; level 4a: evidence is available from clinical case reports; level 4: this represents a consensus of respected experts or expert committees.

Table 15.2: An overview of therapeutic options for pompholyx (based on best available evidence)

	Topical	Systemic	Phototherapy
First line	• Topical corticosteroids • Emollients • Tar-based preparations • Tacrolimus	• Oral antibiotics • Oral antihistamines • Steroids	
Second line		Cyclosporin	a. UVA, PUVA, and narrow band UVB b. Intradermal botulinum A toxin (100 units once) c. Alitretinoin (NA in India)
Third line		• Azathioprine (100–150 mg/d) • Methotrexate (12.5–22.5 mg/wk) • Mycophenolate mofetil (1.5 g/d) • Cyclosporin 3 mg/kg/day for 6 weeks	

*Neomycin based preparations can cause allergic contact dermatitis.

Bibliography

1. Guillet MH, Wierzbicka E, Guillet S, Dagregorio G, Guillet G. A 3-year causative study of pompholyx in 120 patients. Arch Dermatol. 2007; 143(12):1504–8.

2. Storrs F. Acute and recurrent vesicular hand dermatitis not pompholyx or dyshidrosis. Arch Dermatol. 2007;143(12):1578–80.

3. Wollina U. Pompholyx. A review of clinical features, differential diagnosis, and management. Am J Clin Dermatol. 2010;11(5):306–14.

16

Juvenile Plantar Dermatosis

Chapped fissured feet (sweaty sock dermatitis, peridigital dermatitis, juvenile plantar dermatosis).

CLINICAL FEATURES

This is seen initially with scaling, erythema, fissuring, and loss of the epidermal ridge pattern. The tendency to severe chapping declines with age and disappears around the age of puberty. Though most books use the term juvenile plantar dermatoses and some associate it with a atopic tendency, this may not be the case always. The mean age of onset is 7.3 years; the mean age of remission is 14.3 years. Onset is in early fall or when the weather becomes cold and heavy socks and impermeable shoes or boots are worn. An artificial intertrigo is created when moist socks are kept in contact with the soles. The skin in pressure areas, toes, and metatarsal regions becomes dry, brittle, and scaly, and then fissured. The chapping extends onto the sides of the toes. Eventually, the entire sole may be involved; sometimes the hands are also affected. The eruption lasts throughout the winter, clears without treatment in the late spring, and predictably recurs. A common differential is atopic dermatitis of the feet in children which occurs on the dorsal toes and usually not on the plantar surface, and is itchy.

DIFFERENTIAL DIAGNOSIS

The differential diagnosis includes psoriasis, tinea pedis, and allergic contact dermatitis.

Psoriasis: The erythema in psoriasis is darker and the scales in chapped fissured feet are adherent, and removal of the scales causes bleeding.

Fungal infections: Tinea of the feet in children is rare. Feet with the rare case of familial *Trichophyton rubrum* are pale brown and have a fine scale. Fissuring is minimal, and there is little seasonal variation.

Allergic contact dermatitis to shoes usually affects the dorsal aspect and spares the soles, webs, and sides of the feet. The eruption is bright red and scaly rather than pale red and chapped.

TREATMENT

Topical steroids and lubrication provide some relief. Group II or III topical steroids are applied twice each day or, preferably, with plastic wrap occlusion at bedtime. Lubricating creams are applied several times each day, especially directly after removing moist socks to seal in moisture. The feet should not be allowed to remain moist inside shoes. Preventive measures include changing into light leather shoes and changing cotton socks one or two times each day.

Bibliography

1. Eczema, in. Sardana k, Mahajan S, Garg VK. Diagnosis and Management of Skin Disorders: An Evidence-Based Approach, 1/ e.: Lippincott Williams and Wilkins, 2012 (reprint 2015).
2. Fast Facts: Eczema and Contact Dermatitis By John Berth-Jones, Eunice Tan and Howard I Malbach Published 2004.
3. Thieme Clinical Companions Dermatology. Sterry, Dermatology© 2006 Thieme.

17

Venous Eczema

Stasis dermatitis (also known as "Gravitational eczema," "Stasis eczema," and "Varicose eczema") refers to a common form of eczema/dermatitis that affects one or both lower legs in association with venous insufficiency. Insufficient venous return results in increased pressure in the capillaries with the result that both fluid and cells may "leak" out of the capillaries. This results in red cells breaking down, with iron containing hemosiderin possibly contributing to the pathology of this entity.

ETIOLOGY

Stasis dermatitis occurs as a direct consequence of venous insufficiency. Disturbed function of the 1-way valvular system in the deep venous plexus of the legs results in a backflow of blood from the deep venous system to the superficial venous system, with accompanying venous hypertension. This loss of valvular function can result from an age-related decrease in valve competency. This distends the local capillary bed and widens the endothelial pores, thus allowing fibrinogen molecules to escape into the interstitial fluid, where they form a fibrin sheath around the capillaries. This layer of fibrin presumably forms a pericapillary barrier to the diffusion of oxygen and other nutrients which are essential for the normal vitality of the skin. Cutaneous inflammation in venous hypertension may result from increased sequestration of white cells in the venules, with consequent release of proteolytic enzymes and free radicals which produce tissue damage (Fig. 17.1).

Alternatively, specific events, such as deep venous thrombosis, surgery (e.g. vein stripping, total knee arthroplasty, harvesting of saphenous veins for coronary bypass), or traumatic injury, can severely damage the function of the lower extremity venous system (Fig. 17.1).

CLINICAL FEATURES

It is usually seen around the ankle and lower leg. It typically occurs in medial supramalleolar region where microangiopathy is more intense. The eczema may develop suddenly or insidiously. The patients are usually middle-aged or elderly and most often female. The skin appears thin, brown and tissue-like, with possible skin lesions (macule or patches), red spots, superficial skin irritation and/or darkening and/or thickening of the skin at the ankles or legs (Fig. 17.2). The skin may be weakened and may ulcerate in areas. Legs, ankles, or other areas may become swollen. The patient complain of itching, soreness and pains in the legs.

Complications of Stasis Dermatitis

Cellulitis: The cracks and poor skin condition of this disorder predisposes for the entry of bacterial infection causing spreading cellulitis infection in the leg. Crusting or scaling is the most important sign in eczema and this is not seen in cellulitis, where

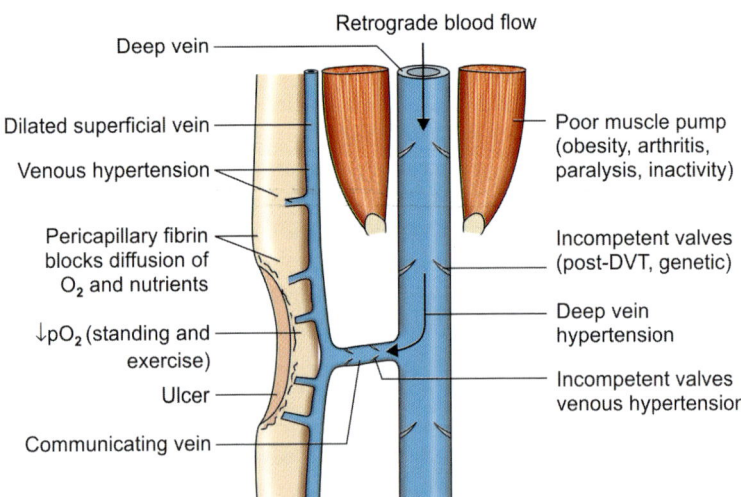

Fig. 17.1: An overview of the factors that determine leg ulcers and venous eczema

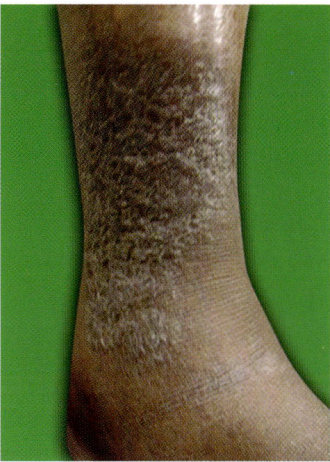

Fig. 17.2: A case of venous eczema with changes of subacute eczema seen on the medial aspect of the limb

the skin is smooth and shiny. Small blisters (vesicles) are common in eczema. These break-down and the serous fluid released dries to form crusts (Fig. 17.2). Although blister formation is uncommon in cellulitis, if blisters do develop they are large and herald the onset of skin necrosis. If the skin condition deteriorates further and breaks down, a venous ulcer (also known as a stasis ulcer) may form.

Lipodermatosclerosis: Stasis dermatitis can lead to fat necrosis with the end stage being permanent sclerosis (lipodermatosclerosis) with inverted champagne bottle appearance. The eczema can also accompanied with small patches of white, atrophic, telangiectatic scarring (atrophie blanche).

Differential Diagnosis

- Atopic dermatitis
- Allergic contact dermatitis
- Discoid eczema
- Infective eczema
- Necrobiosis lipoidica
- Nummular dermatitis
- Pigmented purpuric dermatitis
- Pretibial myxedema

INVESTIGATION

Contact sensitization to active drugs or to their constituents is a continuously operating factor and is one of the factors responsible for the chronicity and deterioration in stasis dermatitis. Patch test should be used to identify the topical agents that may be responsible for perpetuation or aggravation of eczema, especially in patients who do not improve despite adequate treatment of other underlying cause(s). Additionally, it is imperative to consider unprescribed medications causing sudden exacerbation of existing dermatitis.

TREATMENT

The underlying venous hypertension should be controlled. Obese patients should be urged to lose weight. Well-fitted support stockings or firm bandages can be helpful if worn regularly and care is taken to avoid the formation of a band at the top of the leg. The legs should be elevated as effectively as possible. Mild topical steroids may be used to relieve irritation, but the use of potent steroids should be limited to short periods of a few days as they may cause cutaneous atrophy and increase the risk of ulceration. Topical tacrolimus has been reported to be effective. Bacterial infection must be treated where appropriate, but the risk of sensitization to topical antibiotics and antiseptics should be borne in mind, and systemic antibiotics may be preferable. If trauma is thought to be playing a part, and the patient cannot resist scratching, a bandage may be helpful. Aspirin (300 mg per day) and pentoxifylline may improve healing of venous ulcer.

Venous disease is progressive and irreversible. Patient must be educated about the need for continual hemodynamic support. It is a mistake to place compression stocking on edematous limbs, especially if they are tender. One should use compression bandaging until all edema, tenderness and inflammation have resolved.

Bibliography

1. Eczema, in. Sardana k, Mahajan S, Garg VK. Diagnosis and Management of Skin Disorders: An Evidence-Based Approach, 1/ e.: Lippincott Williams and Wilkins, 2012 (reprint 2015).
2. Fast Facts: Eczema and Contact Dermatitis By John Berth-Jones, Eunice Tan and Howard I Malbach Published 2004.
3. Thieme Clinical Companions Dermatology. Sterry, Dermatology© 2006 Thieme.

18

Lichen Simplex Chronicus

This is a self-inflicting dermatoses which is seen in patients with high stress levels and some clinicians believe that the patients derive pleasure from itching and is possibly a stress reliever.

CLINICAL FEATURES

It is perpetuated by constant scratching and rubbing . The lesions are seen on sites accessible by the dominant hand and are characterized by very thick oval plaques with a persistent course or with frequent recurrences (Figs 18.1 to 18.3). Occasionally they may be bilateral (Fig. 18.4). As most patients derive great pleasure

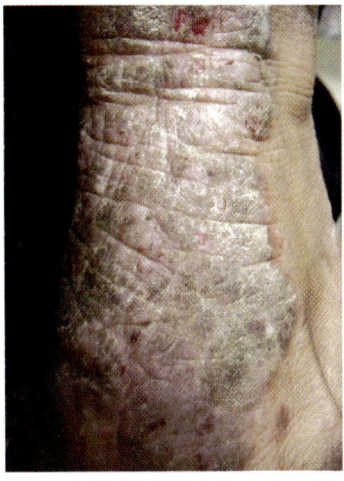

Fig. 18.1: A plaque of lichen simplex chronicus on the back of the foot. Note the thickened and lichenified skin

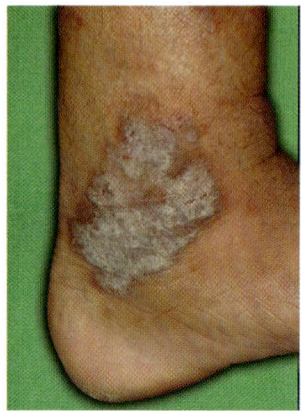

Fig. 18.2: Side of the ankle is a common site of this dermatoses and patients often use blunt objects to scratch these areas

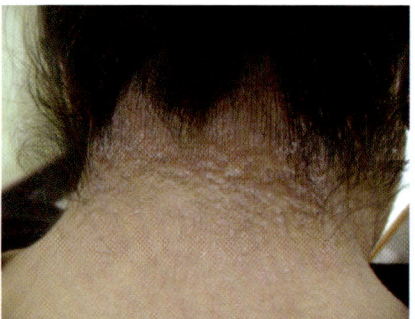

Fig. 18.3: Initial stage of lichen simplex nuchae on the neck in a female patient

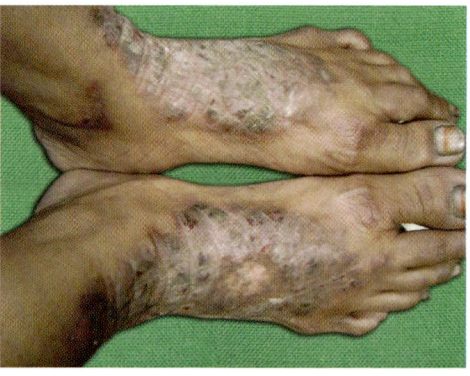

Fig. 18.4: Bilateral lichen simplex chronicus

in the relief that comes from frantically scratching the inflamed site, this is habit forming dermatoses has frequent recurrences. The individual lesion is a thickened like a bark of the tree with accentuation of skin lines (lichenification) (Fig. 18.1). The sites of involvement often conform to the reach of the dominant hand (Box 18.1) (Figs 18.5 and 18.6).

Box 18.1: Sites of involvement of lichen simplex chronicus

Outer lower portion of lower leg

Genital: Scrotum, vulva, anal area, pubis

Wrists and ankles (Figs 18.1 and 18.2)

Upper eyelids

Back (lichen simplex nuchae) and side of neck (Fig. 18.3)

Orifice of the ear

Extensor forearms near elbow

Fold behind the ear

Scalp (Picker's nodules)

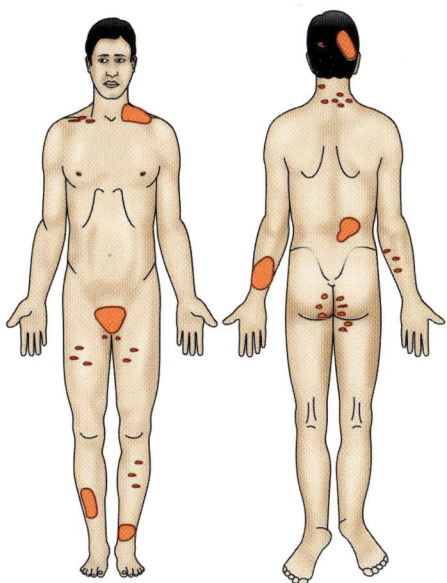

Fig. 18.5: Sites of involvement in lichen simplex chronicus

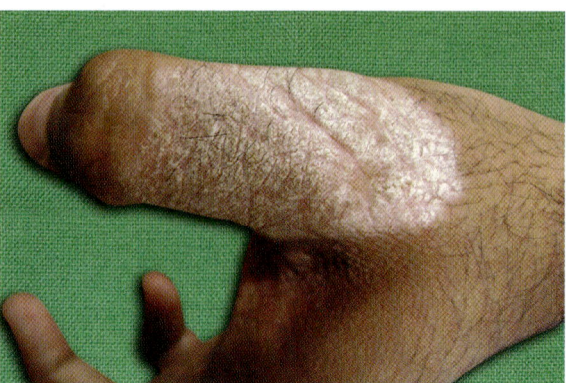

Fig. 18.6: An unusual site of lichen simplex chronicus, here the patient used to rub the finger on the side of a table

TREATMENT

The patient must be, made to understand that the rash will not clear until even minor scratching and rubbing are stopped, but in most cases this is a habitual tendency and most patients cannot stop the tendency to scratch. Scratching frequently takes place during sleep, and the affected area may have to be covered to word this trauma.

The fundamentals of treatment are outlined in the introduction section on eczematous inflammation. Clobetasol foams (not available in India) are very effective and can be used for lesions on the neck, legs, wrists, ankles, and vulva. Treatment of the anal area or the fold behind the ear does not require potent topical steroids as do other forms of lichen simplex and groups V or VI topical steroids suffice. *Lichen simplex nuchae* (Fig. 18.3), because of its location, is difficult to treat. Inflammation that extends into the scalp may be treated with a group II steroid gel. Moist, secondarily infected areas respond to oral antibiotics and topical steroid solutions (e.g. clobetasol solution). A 2- to 3-week course of prednisone (20 mg twice daily) should be considered when an extensively inflamed scalp does not respond rapidly to topical treatment. Nodules may require monthly intralesional injections with triamcinolone acetonide (kenalog 10 mg/ml). Botulinum A toxin injected intradermally into lichenified lesions may block acetylcholine release and control pruritus. An evidence based tabulation of treatment options given are in Table 18.1.

Table 18.1: An overview of therapeutic options for lichen simplex chronicus

	Topical	Systemic	Other options
First line	• Topical corticosteroids • IL Steroids	Oral antihistamines	
Second line	• Tacrolimus • Doxepin (NA in India) • Capsaicin		
Third line		• Ketotifen (1 mg BD) • Aspirin • Gabapentin (300 mg/day increased by 300 mg/day every 3 days to a final dose of 900 mg/day) • Botulinum toxin (20 units of botulinum toxin type A (100 U/ml) per 2 cm × 2 cm area of an LSC plaque).	• Transcutaneous electrical stimulation • Acupuncture and electroacupuncture • Psychotherapy • Hypnosis • Psychopharmacotherapy • Surgical excision

Bibliography

1. Eczema, in. Sardana k, Mahajan S, Garg VK. Diagnosis and Management of Skin Disorders: An Evidence-Based Approach, 1/e.: Lippincott Williams and Wilkins, 2012 (reprint 2015).
2. Fast Facts: Eczema and Contact Dermatitis By John Berth-Jones, Eunice Tan and Howard I Malbach Published 2004.
3. Thieme Clinical Companions Dermatology. Sterry, Dermatology© 2006 Thieme.

19

Exfoliative Erythroderma

Though erythroderma, the commonly used parlance of the above stated disorder, is uncommon, this is a condition that is best managed by an inpatient facility as the disease has a long remitting and relapsing course and may need good nursing care.

CLINICAL FEATURES

Clinically it is characterized by an involvement of more than 80% of the BSA with erythema and scaling (Fig. 19.1) and though there are clinical signs described to determine the etiology, in most cases they are not reliable and this entity is best described as a clinical phenotype.

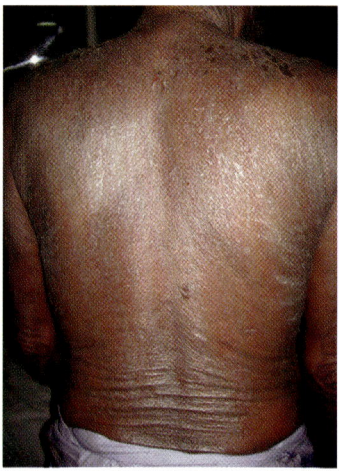

Fig. 19.1: Diffuse involvement of the skin with erythema and scaling

Erythroderma is thus a clinical state that results from a variety of specific dermatologic disorders, including psoriasis, pityriasis rubra pilaris, contact dermatitis, atopic dermatitis, drug reactions, and cutaneous T-cell lymphoma, as well as underlying malignancies. Specific therapy requires the proper diagnosis (Fig. 19.2) but all erythrodermas may initially be treated in a similar manner. The initial therapeutic strategy is control of symptoms and prevention of the complications of erythroderma (fluid and calorie loss, heat loss, weight loss). Specific treatment must be tailored to the disease causing the erythroderma.

TREATMENT

Hospitalization or admission to a day skin treatment center should be considered, as an aggressive topical approach can be too complex and demanding for a home care plan. Elderly patients are at risk for significant medical complications, including high output cardiac failure, septicemia, hypothermia, pneumonia, and anemia. Unless the underlying diagnosis is known, initial treatment is usually topical and should include the following:

General Advise

1. A warm, humid environment, and blankets to stop shivering.
2. Soaking in warm water followed by a bland emollient is a useful adjunct.
3. After each bath, application of a medium-potency steroid in a preservative-free ointment (triamcinolone ointment 0.1%) to the whole affected surface.
4. Hydroxyzine 25–50 mg orally for control of itch and sedation.
5. A high-protein diet with B vitamins, iron supplementation, and adequate nutrition, and correction of any fluid or electrolyte imbalance are essential in this catabolic state.
6. Discontinuation of all unnecessary systemic drugs is prudent if drug induced erythroderma is a possible diagnosis.

Other Measures

1. Antibiotics are recommended by some, but are not generally necessary unless secondary infection is present.
2. Systemic corticosteroids may be employed in cases of refractory drug-induced or idiopathic but *not psoriatic erythroderma*. Initial

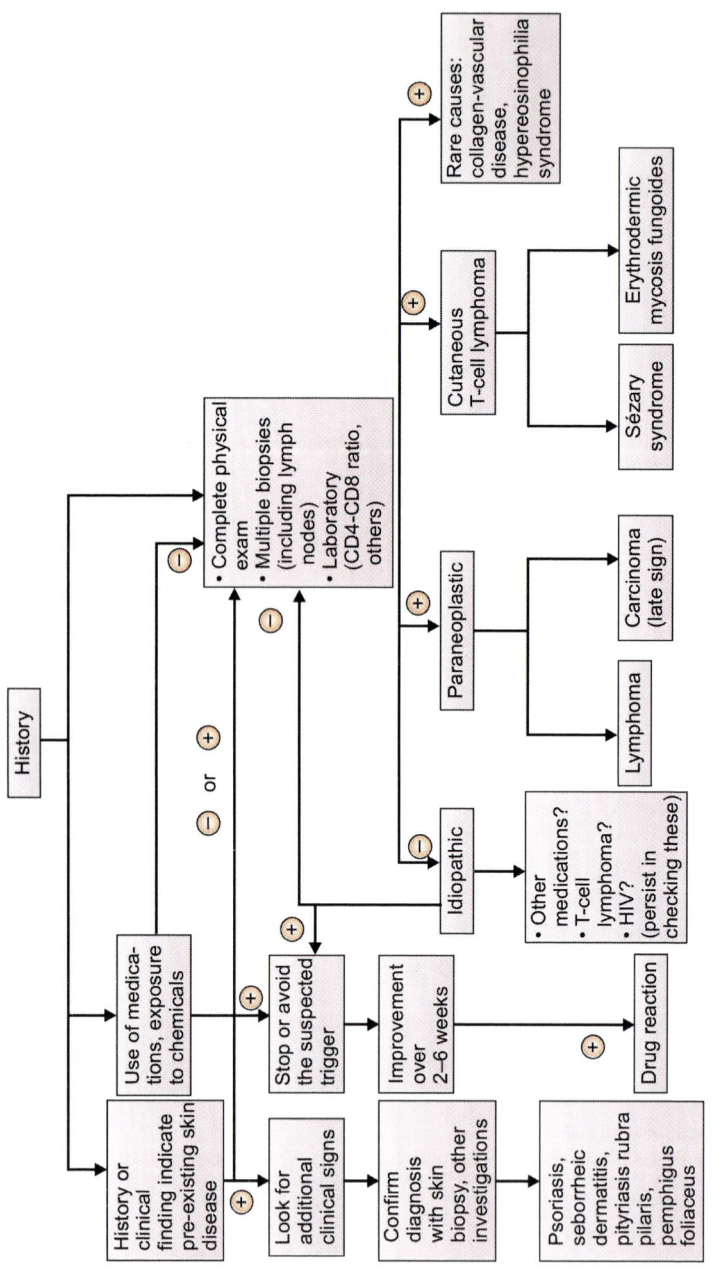

Fig. 19.2: A proposed method of identifying the likley cause of erythroderma

dose of prednisone 1 to 3 mg/kg/day is a reasonable start and should be rapidly tapered when clearing is achieved.

3. Cyclosporin has also been employed in refractory, idiopathic and psoriatic patients. Initial dosage of 5 mg/kg/day with subsequent reduction to 1–3 mg/kg/day are appropriate.

Bibliography

1. Eczema, in. Sardana k, Mahajan S, Garg VK. Diagnosis and Management of Skin Disorders: An Evidence-Based Approach, 1/ e.: Lippincott Williams and Wilkins, 2012 (reprint 2015).

2. Fast Facts: Eczema and Contact Dermatitis By John Berth-Jones, Eunice Tan and Howard I Malbach Published 2004.

3. Thieme Clinical Companions Dermatology. Sterry, Dermatology© 2006 Thieme.

20

Prurigo Nodularis

INTRODUCTION

Prurigo nodularis (PN) is a chronic relapsing, highly pruritic condition characterized by the presence of hyperkeratotic, excoriated, pruritic papules and nodules, with a tendency to symmetrical distribution. This condition is a difficult disease to treat and causes frustration to both the patient and the treating doctor. It has a high impact on the quality of life of the patient.

Incidence and prevalence of PN in the general population are unknown, because in epidemiological studies, PN is often listed under chronic itchy disorders (Iking A). In female patients PN seems to be more prevalent, to occur at an earlier age, and to be more severe than in male patients. Individuals with PN can be divided into those who are atopic or nonatopic. In the setting of atopy, PN has an earlier age of onset and may be accompanied by cutaneous hypersensitivity to various environmental allergens.

Etiopathogenesis

The etiology is poorly understandable. The most common dermatological disorder associated to PN is atopic dermatitis, described also as 'atopic prurigo' (Pugliarello S). Systemic diseases frequently associated PN are type 2 diabetes mellitus, thyroid disorders, HCV infection, non-Hodgkin lymphoma and psychiatric disorders, particularly depression and anxiety (Winhoven SM). In some cases, no underlying disease is detected (idiopathic PN).

The pathogenesis of PN is still unknown; however, recent findings suggest that PN might be consequent to chronic itch induced by neuropathy (Yosipovitch G). A distinctive characteristic of neuropathic itch is the co-existence of other sensory symptoms as paresthesia, hyperesthesia or hypoesthesia, as well as burning, tingling, stinging and heat and cold sensations. Nerve growth factor has been implicated in the pathogenesis of prurigo nodularis. Calcitonin gene-related peptide and substance P immunoreactive nerves are markedly increased in prurigo nodularis when compared with normal skin.

Clinical Features

The classic lesion in PN is a firm pruritic nodule that is hyperkeratotic a the lensions numbers from a few to hundreds, and ranges from several millimeters to 2 cm in diameter (Fig. 20.1). There is a tendency for symmetrical distribution, with a predilection for extensor surfaces of the limbs; however, the trunk may be involved. The face and palms are seldom affected although no part of the body is exempt. Sparing of the upper mid back, known as 'butterfly sign', is distinctive. Prominent features include crusting and excoriations with post inflammatory hyperpigmented and hypopigmented macules (Fig. 20.2). The skin between the lesions is usually normal but can be xerotic or lichenified.

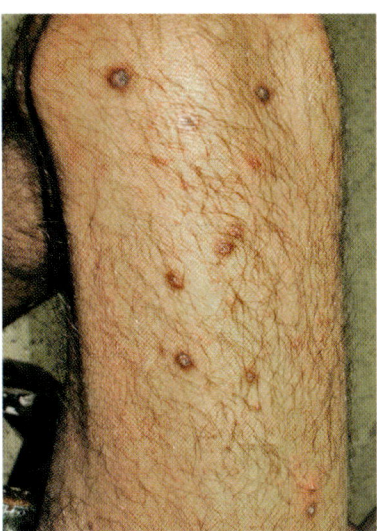

Fig. 20.1: Multipe, hyperkeratotic, nodules, with some showing excoriation and crusting on the leg in a male patient

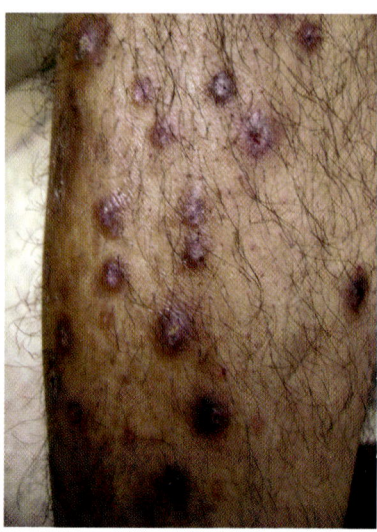

Fig. 20.2: Excoriated papules, with some lesions healing with post-inflammatory hyperpigmentation

Investigations

An important first step in therapy is to identify any underlying associations and treat accordingly. Table 20.1 lists the suggested investigations for these underlying associations (Lee MR).

Table 20.1: Suggested investigations for associated disorders in prurigo nodularis

Full blood count
Liver function test
Urea, creatinine, electrolytes
Parathyroid hormone level
Thyroid function test
Hepatitis serology
HIV serology
Total serum IgE level
Tuberculin test: Skin biopsy for
Histopathology
Direct immunofluorence
Indirect immunofluorence
Patch testing

Treatment

Treatment of PN is still a challenge, and it is frustrating for both dermatologists and patients because, in the majority of cases, the response is limited and unsatisfactory. Once the itch–scratch cycle 'takes over', it is extremely difficult to stop. There is no standardized therapy of PN, and evidence from RCT is limited. Treatments include topical, systemic and physical approaches. Table 20.2 outlines the topical and systemic treatments currently used for PN (Lee MR).

Table 20.2: Current treatments available for prurigo nodularis

Topical antipruritics: Menthol and phenol
Oral antihistamines: Promethazine hydrochloride
Oral tricyclic antidepressants: Doxepin
Topical and intralesional glucocorticoids
Narrow-band UV B, and PUVA
Cryotherapy
Topical vitamin D
Capsaicin
Cyclosporin
Thalidomide
Laser
Naltrexone

General Measures

Simple measures such as clipping the fingernails and recommending the use of gloves or mittens can be helpful. It is important to stress to the patient the requirement to apply emollients as xerosis usually worsens the pruritus.

First-line Agents

Topical antipruritics such as 1% menthol or phenol in a creamy base may be used to reduce the itch. Oral antihistamines such as promethazine hydrochloride 25–75 mg at night, or oral antidepressants such as doxepin 10–75 mg at night may be administered to reduce the pruritus. Potent topical glucocorticoid creams or ointments, such as betamethasone dipropionate 0.5 mg/g, glucocorticoid creams under occlusion, and intralesional glucocorticoids, such as triamcinolone acetonide 10 mg/ml increasing to 40 mg/ml suspension, are often employed. Occlusive bandages are useful as they interrupt the itch–scratch cycle.

Second-line Agents

UV light exposure has been shown to lessen the pruritus and can be beneficial in the treatment of PN. The main effect of UV light treatment in PN is to break the cycle of itching and scratching. Cryotherapy is a useful therapeutic agent for the treatment of PN. It can also be combined with intralesional corticosteroids.

Recently, topical *vitamin D₃* has been reported to be effective in the treatment of PN. Vitamin D_3 down regulates cellular adhesion molecule expression by inhibiting TNF-α mRNA expression. Capsaicin has been shown to reduce pruritus and induce complete disappearance of lesions. When applied topically it induces itch and a burning sensation as well as erythema.

Third-line Agents

Cyclosporin has demonstrated unequivocal improvement of PN as well as a reduction in the severity of pruritus. Cyclosporin inhibits lymphokine transcription and lymphocyte activation and proliferation.

The first reported use of *thalidomide* in the treatment of PN was in 1975. Thalidomide inhibits polymorphonuclear leukocyte chemotaxis and selectively inhibits TNF-α production by enhancing degradation of TNF-α mRNA. It has been postulated that thalidomide causes central nervous system depression without causing incoordination, respiratory depression or narcosis. Through its central sedative effect, it causes a decreased perception of peripheral stimuli. Thalidomide may have a direct peripheral action on the proliferated neural tissue in the lesions causing PN. There have been reported cases where oral thalidomide at doses of 200 mg daily demonstrated improvement of pruritus and flattening of lesions with no serious adverse events.

Naltrexone has been reported to have a high antipruritic effect in patients with PN. Opiates have been shown to evoke or potentiate itch, independently from their histamine-releasing effect. *Gabapentin*, *pregabalin* and the neurokinin receptor 1 antagonist, *aprepitant*, seem also to be effective in the therapy of PN, but RCTs are still lacking (Fostini AC).

Most likely, patients with PN need to be approached with combination therapy, which includes suppression of multiple mediators, including cytokines and neuromediators.

Bibliography

1. Fostini AC, Girolomoni G, Tessari G. Prurigo nodularis: an update on etiopathogenesis and therapy. J Dermatolog Treat 2013 Dec;24(6):458–62.
2. Iking A, Grundmann S, Chatzigeorgakidis E, Phan NQ, Klein D, Ständer S. Prurigo as a symptom of atopic and non-atopic diseases: aetiological survey in a consecutive cohort of 108 patients. J Eur Acad Dermatol Venereol 2013;27:550–7.
3. Lee MR, Shumack S. Prurigo nodularis: a review. Australas J Dermatol 2005 Nov;46(4):211–18.
4. Pugliarello S, Cozzi A, Gisondi P, Girolomoni G. Phenotypes of atopic dermatitis. J Dtsch Dermatol Ges 2011;9:12–20.
5. Winhoven SM, Gawkrodger DJ. Nodular prurigo: metabolic diseases are a common association. Clin Exp Dermatol 2007;32:224–225.
6. Yosipovitch G, Samuel LS. Neuropathic and psychogenic itch. Dermatol Ther 2008;21.32–41.

Index

A (PUVA) 118
Acute 1, 3
Airborne 56
Alba, pityriasis 114
Alitretinoin 132
Amiantacea, pityriasis 99
Atopic 122
Aureus, Staphylococcus 80
Axilla 27
Azathioprine 132

Barrier-protectant 13
Bathes, bleach 93
Botulinum 131
Burow 4

Cataracts 88
CD, irritant 9
Cellulitis 146
Cement 4, 61
Chromate 28
Chronic 1
Cobalt 17
Contact, irritant dermatitis 8
Contact, pigmented dermatitis 40
Corticosteroids 4, 131
Cosmetic, pigmented dermatitis 41
Cyclosporine 132

Dermatitis 1
    atopic 11, 77
    contact 17
    diaper 68
    seborrheic 98
    stasis 145

Diaper 15
Dichromate 120
Dichromate, potassium 17
Discoid 125
Dye, hair 3

Eczema
    apron 126
    craqueli 107
    discoid 109
    fingertip 126
    hyperkeratotic 134
    nipple 86
    papular 81
    ring 126
    venous 145
Eczemas 1
Exfoliativa, keratolysis 127
Eyelid 26

Filaggrin 79
Fingertip 15
Fold, Dennie-Morgan 85
Foot 29
Formaldehyde 17, 120
Fragrance 17
Fragrances 120

Hand 25
Herpeticum, eczema 88
Housewives 9
Hybrid 122
Hyperkeratotic 6, 124
Hypothesis, hygiene 78

IgE, serum levels 89
Infantum, gluteale 68
Intralesional 7
Irritant 8

Jacquet 68

Keratoconjunctivitis 88
Keratolytics 130

Lanolin 120
Laser 118
Leiner 99
Lichenification 77, 151
Lichenoid 40
    frictional eruption 86
Lick, lip 9, 13
Lip-licker 85
Lipodermatosclerosis 147
Lobe, ear 26
Lymphomatoid 45

Malassezia 80, 99
Melanosis, Riehl 40
Methotrexate 132
Mirror-image 110
Moisturizers 130
Multiforme, erythema 39
Mupirocin 93

Neck 27
Nickel 17, 120
Nodules, Picker 150

Palmar, hyperkeratotic 11
Palms, hyperlinear 79
Paraben 17
Parthenium 56
Perioral 26
Photoallergic 30
Phototherapy 93, 131, 137
Pilaris, keratosis 79, 86

Pimecrolimus 131
Plantar, juvenile dermatosis 86
Pollens 56
Pompholyx 123
Potassium 120
P-phenylenediamine 21, 29
Protein 122
Prurigo nodularis 81
Psoriasis 11
Purpuric 39
Pustular 45

RAST 89
Repair, barrier 91
Retinoids 131
Ring 14
Rubber 40, 120

Sawdust 60
Scalp 29
Sign, Hertoghe 86
Simplex
    lichen chronicus 149
    lichen nuchae 150
SLS 9
Spongiosis 1
Steroids 92, 130
Subacute 1

Tacrolimus 5, 118, 131
Tar, coal 131
Textile 40
Th1 79
Th2 79
Tinea 11
Triangle, Wilkinson 30
Trunk 27

Vulgaris, ichthyosis 79

Wear and tear 15, 124